HAVE HEALTHY TEETH AND GUMS

HAVE HEALTHY TEETH AND GUMS

**MERVYN PICHEL
AND NEIL CURTIS**

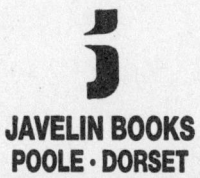

**JAVELIN BOOKS
POOLE · DORSET**

First published in the UK 1986 by Javelin Books,
Link House, West Street, Poole, Dorset, BH15 1LL

Distributed in the United States by
Sterling Publishing Co., Inc.,
2 Park Avenue, New York, NY 10016

British Library Cataloguing in Publication Data

Pichel, Mervyn
  Have healthy teeth and gums.
  1. Teeth—Care and hygiene
  I. Title   II. Curtis, Neil
  617.6'01   RK61

ISBN 0 7137 1431 X

Typeset in 9/10½ point Baskerville by
Nene Phototypesetters Ltd, Northampton

Printed in Great Britain by
Hazell Watson & Viney Limited,
Member of the BPCC Group,
Aylesbury, Bucks.

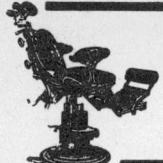

CONTENTS

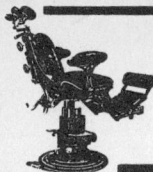

AUTHOR'S PREFACE

The idea for this book first entered my head in 1972. After realizing that many people prefer to discuss dentistry well away from the surgery, I decided to make some notes on some of the more commonly asked questions. Within twelve months, there were, perhaps, enough ideas to make several volumes but, surprisingly at that time, there seemed to be few publishers interested in such a proposal. With a greater public awareness of 'whole body health', however, the task of finding a publisher became much easier. But, writing style and dental research and practice do not always go hand in hand and my chance meeting with Neil Curtis became a turning point in the eventual acceptance and publication of this book. He, as a non-dental author, 'humanized' the book and finally contributed to the text. I am particularly·pleased that he did so because the book is for patients, not dentists. Neil Curtis is editorial director of Curtis Garratt Limited and has been instrumental in the publication of many books. In one of his books he even made spiders sound attractive! My sincere thanks to him for his encouragement and patience.

I should like also to acknowledge the contribution of all who work in dental research. Many of the factual statements made in this book come, I know, from painstaking research carried out by a large number of people.

Finally, my thanks to the many people who have read various tracts of the text and, in particular, my especial gratitude to my wife, Gillian, for reading over the words several dozen times during the last six years.

Mervyn Pichel
Oxford, 1986

7

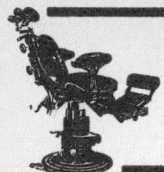

ACKNOWLEDGEMENTS

The authors wish to acknowledge the assistance of the following people in producing this book:

Catherine Barrow of Stafford Miller Products for providing the information on fluoride supplementation.

Dr S. Joyston-Bechal for giving so generously of her time to advise on the difficult subject of fluoridation and fluoride supplementation in particular. We are also indebted to Dr Joyston-Bechal and T. B. Dowell for allowing us to reproduce the Fluoride Supplement Dosage Chart which appeared in the *British Dental Journal* in 1981: No. 150, pages 273–75. We also acknowledge permission to reproduce this article and to refer to the *British Dental Journal* elsewhere in the text.

Thanks are due to Tom Birch for giving some preliminary dental photography lessons to the authors.

We also acknowledge the faith shown in our book by the publishers, Blandford Press.

We owe thanks to Mr Richard Fieldhouse, Dip Orth, RCS for allowing us to use study models to produce the photograph number 20.

The General Dental Council kindly granted permission for us to quote from the 'Notice for the Guidance of Dentists', November 1981, relating to the administration of sedatives and anaesthetics by dental surgeons.

Hamilton Photographic Services made the difficult task of photographing X-ray pictures much easier than we could have managed unaided due to their expertise at their High Wycombe studio. Our thanks and praises also to Mr R. Higham, of Keen Commercial Photographic, High Wycombe for producing such excellent photographs.

Our sincere thanks also to Lawrence Kotlow, DDS for his kind letter of encouragement and for allowing us to refer to his article on breast feeding as it appeared in the *American Journal of Dentistry for Children* May 1977, pages 192–3. Also from the USA, we thank the American Society for Clinical Nutrition for permission to produce the Comparison Table of

Human and Cow's Milk as it appeared in the *American Journal of Clinical Nutrition*, 24 Aug., 1971, page 971, Gyorgy & Paul.

We acknowledge the assistance given to us by the Pharmaceutical Press and the courtesy of Her Majesty's Stationery Office in allowing us to reproduce the 'Steroid Warning Card' (Crown Copyright).

Our thanks also to Miss A. E. Welham of Johnson and Johnson Dental Division at Slough, Buckinghamshire for kindly arranging the drawings in *Figure 9*. We thank the photographic department of Johnson and Johnson for their work on our behalf, too.

To Richard Satherley our grateful thanks for allowing us to use his photographs to show 'a glimpse of the future' in the photograph in the eight-page photo section.

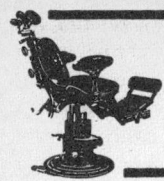

INTRODUCTION

'I'm certainly not going back to the dentist again until I have to. I haven't been for ten years and now she tells me that I have to have thirteen fillings.' This records, as accurately as memory will allow, part of a conversation between two young ladies, overheard during the course of a train journey. Sadly, it reflects the fears that 'going to the dentist' still hold for many people despite health education programmes and the advances that have been made in dental science in recent years. Too many people still seem willing to suffer the pain and inconvenience of the loss of some or all of their own teeth by middle age, or even much earlier, either from neglect or an unwillingness to visit the dentist regularly. It is the aim of this book to convince everyone that tooth decay is not an inevitable consequence of normal living and that they, together with their dentist, can do much to ensure that their teeth and gums will stay healthy and look good for most if not all of their lives.

Many of us lavish more attention and money on our motor cars than we are prepared to expend on our teeth. Although it is possible to buy a brand new car, a new mouth cannot easily be purchased – at least, not one that is as good as the one we are born with! Apart from those of the human species, the teeth of most animals last their lifetime although, of course, in most cases, this is rather shorter than the traditional 'three score years and ten' and, in many instances, it is tooth loss or tooth wear which determines the animal's fate when it is no longer able to feed. Ironically, it has been our own ingenuity which has, to some extent, led to the all too common neglect of our teeth. We have been able to cut, prepare, and cook our food so that loss of teeth did not lead to starvation, even before the advent of the aid much loved by the stand-up comic, the denture!

In the wild, animals rely on their teeth for a variety of activities including killing prey, tearing up and masticating all kinds of different food items, defence, locomotion, grooming, and communication through facial expressions. Some animals even use their teeth to hold on to a mate! It is also true that, generally, few animals, apart from ourselves, have access to the kinds of food and drinks, such as sweets, candies and fizzy 'pop', that lead so quickly to tooth decay although every pet owner knows that a dog will soon become addicted to chocolate if it is offered as a treat. On the other hand, animals are obliged to deal with tough grasses or even bones when they eat so their teeth may easily be worn down. But wildlife conservationists would find their task even harder than it is if animals faced tooth decay and gum disease on the same scale as civilized human beings.

It was almost 100 years ago that Arthur Ebbles wrote in the scientific journal, *Nature*, 'There is little doubt that an open air life and healthy surroundings encourage the formation of sound teeth in a sound body; but I cannot but think that the principal cause of caries (tooth decay) must be looked for in the food.' He went on to say that imperfect nutrition during the development of the teeth (i.e. from conception), together with the use of soft cooked foods, provide some of the factors necessary for the process of decay to begin. We consider ourselves to be at the acme of the evolutionary tree and yet, even though science has known much about the care of teeth since the nineteenth century, it has only been over the last fifteen years or so that public awareness of its importance has been widespread. But still some people seem unable to master the techniques of brushing their teeth, still children are given sweets as a treat rather than nuts or a piece of cheese, and still many are unwilling to visit the dentist and even some that do become hysterical in the waiting room. And so, eight decades after Arthur Ebbles' article in *Nature*, the President of the USA with the famous 'peanut' smile found it necessary to write to the American Dental Society for Children, 'Dental health is a priority concern for all nations; as a parent, I know the critical importance of good dental care to the well-being of a child.'

It is encouraging that tooth decay and gum disease are preventable and that, by easy steps, everyone can have a healthy mouth which will stay healthy:

1   Read this book! It will allay many of your fears.
2   Visit your dentist regularly – you may even look forward to the chat!
3   Clean your teeth and gums regularly and efficiently – this book will help you learn how.
4   Work out and stick to a sound and healthy diet – not just for the sake of your teeth and gums!
5   Make sure your children follow these guidelines.

Perhaps tooth decay and gum disease will one day cease to be two of the commonest diseases in the world.

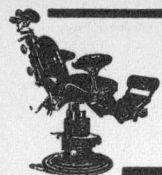

1 THE TEETH AND GUMS, TEETHING, AND THE JAW JOINT

The shape and structure of the human teeth and jaws have evolved over many thousands of years. There are features in our dentition which are reminders of a past when we only ate vegetables as well as characteristics which are more reminiscent of the teeth of meat-eating animals, the carnivores. Over hundreds of thousands of years the bone and gum which support the dentition have also become modified to the form which we see in people today.

A house is only as strong as the foundations upon which it is laid and, similarly, the dentition is dependent upon its supporting structures. If we are to understand better how dental disease can occur and how it can be prevented, it is important that we should have a detailed knowledge of the teeth and gums. Therefore, this chapter takes a relatively comprehensive look at the make-up of the teeth, gums, and jaws and, although it is not intended to be a textbook, its approach does include information that is not normally included in standard dental health education publications.

The teeth begin to form in the human embryo within the first weeks after conception when it is only about six weeks old. At this stage, the whole embryo is only about a centimetre (0.4 inch) long. Clearly, much of the nourishment which is required by the developing child comes directly from the mother so that her diet is of great importance if it is to grow healthily. The newly growing teeth are referred to as 'tooth buds' and there are spaces between each one during the life of the foetus. As the teeth develop, so do the jaws, and, at birth, the lower jaw is perfectly shaped with the exception that the pronounced chin region has not yet formed. If you examine a baby's face closely, you will see that the vertical part of the jaw bone is shorter than it is in an adult. As the teeth move through the bone, or erupt, the jaw bone begins to change. The bony arches of the jaws develop and this is stimulated further by suckling and by tongue and lip movements. This is just one of the reasons why some members of the medical and dental professions encourage breast feeding. The teat on an artificial feeder does not work in the same way as a

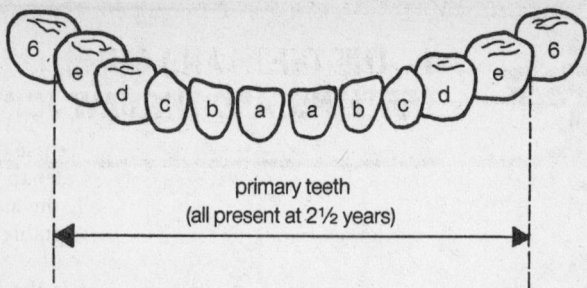

primary teeth
(all present at 2½ years)

Fig. 1 The first of the adult molars appearing behind the last of the primary molars. Note that the first molar (6) of the second dentition appears behind the 'e' of the first dentition. Make sure that your child is aware of the newcomer and remember '6s at six years' – two in the lower jaw and two in the upper jaw.

human nipple although a consultant paediatrician has designed a teat which is closer in function to a human nipple than any other feeder currently used.

In all, twenty teeth erupt between the ages of six months and two-and-a-half years with ten in the upper jaw and ten in the lower. We have mentioned these average dates of eruption, only as a guide. *(See Table 1 on p.136.)* The premature appearance of a tooth does not portend advanced development, nor should you think that a delay in the eruption of teeth indicates that the child is backward or underdeveloped. The condition in which teeth are absent altogether is called 'anodontia' and is distressing for child and parent alike. While anodontia is rare, partial anodontia is quite common and, in some adults, the lateral incisor teeth are often absent.

The first teeth are extremely important in establishing the growth patterns in the face although many other factors come into play, too. Thus, it is vital that you make sure your child's first teeth are well cared for because, if they are lost prematurely through decay or accident, this may cause problems of spacing when the second teeth begin to appear. The first of the permanent teeth, conveniently numbered six in the dental arch, normally erupt after the child's sixth birthday *(see Figure 1)*. Make sure you take note of the presence of this tooth and that the child is aware of the newcomer, too. If it is lost, a permanent tooth will not be replaced naturally. The surface of this tooth is often deeply pitted and fissured so that bacteria can lodge here. Between the ages of six and fourteen, the entire first dentition is replaced by a second or permanent set of teeth. The full complement of second teeth numbers thirty-two but this includes the four wisdom teeth, each of which is number eight in each arch, and these do not normally appear until after the eighteenth birthday.

When they are lost naturally, the first teeth literally fall out because their roots resorb and the tooth loses its attachment to the surrounding structures. It is possible that some of their permanent successors may erupt while the first teeth are still present and this may give rise to some concern because the mouth looks so crowded. Dentists refer to this as 'the ugly duckling' stage but, as the first teeth are shed, the situation improves and the child's appearance becomes more acceptable to the anxious parents.

The first part of the tooth to appear through the gum is the enamel which is the hardest tissue produced in the human body and covers that part of the tooth above gum level. At the tip of the tooth, the enamel is about 2.5 millimetres (1/10 inch) thick and it becomes thinner towards the neck of the tooth at gum level. Everyone knows that the colour of teeth can vary and this is essentially dependent upon the thickness of the enamel *(see Figure 2)*. Where the enamel is thin the underlying dentine *(see below)*, which is a yellowish colour, shows through and the tooth appears to be yellow. At the tip of the tooth where light shines through the enamel, it appears to be an almost bluish-white colour because there is no dentine present at this point. If teeth are very white in colour, it does not necessarily mean that they are any stronger, nor does it suggest that they are more likely to suffer from decay if they are yellowish. Teeth may become stained for a variety of reasons, including from any drugs that a mother may take while she is pregnant, or from those taken during childhood. Even childhood illnesses may affect the appearance of the enamel *(see Chapter 8)*.

Enamel is composed of crystals of a chemical substance called calcium hydroxy apatite. Individual crystals are invisible to the naked eye and the actual crystalline structure of enamel can only be observed using a high-powered electron microscope. The following substances are also present in human tooth enamel: sodium, magnesium, carbonates, and phosphates. Interestingly, the surface of the enamel is richer in fluoride than the rest of the tooth. Fluoride *(see Chapter 2)* is known to inhibit the progress of tooth decay and provides valuable additional protection against tooth-decaying acids which form in the mouth, particularly after eating foods that are high in sucrose.

Beneath the enamel, making up the main 'body' of the tooth, is the dentine, which is yellowish in colour and not so hard as the enamel. Dentine also contains calcium hydroxy apatite crystals, although these are smaller than those found in the enamel. About three-quarters of the dentine by weight is made up of these crystals, while the rest is referred to as the organic content. Research is still being conducted into the

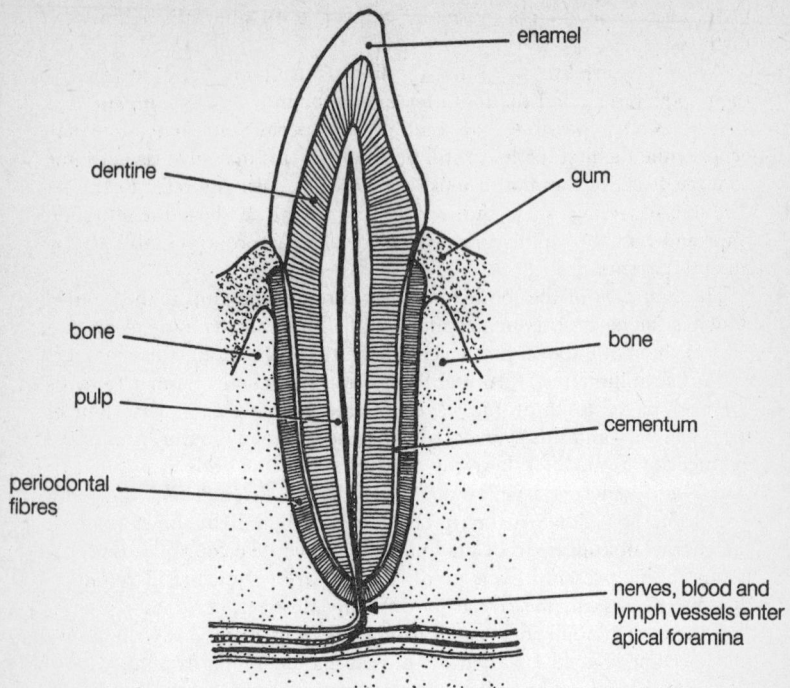

Fig. 2 Diagrammatic section through an incisor tooth and its supporting structures.

structure of dentine, and it is still not fully understood why it is so sensitive. The organic part of the dentine is produced by special cells called *odontoblasts*. They send out long projections or processes which enter the so-called *dentinal tubules* and it is possible that any variations of temperature and pressure on the teeth initiate painful stimuli in these projections which, in turn, are transmitted to the central nerve in the tooth which lies, with its associated blood vessels, in the pulp canal. The nerves and blood vessels which supply a tooth are branches of the major ones shown in Figure 2.

It is these nerves and blood vessels which make up the pulp of the tooth. Inside the pulp canal and pulp chamber, there are also special defence cells which combat infecting bacteria and other microorganisms. The nerves which supply the pulp are two types: one type initiates contraction and expansion of the muscle walls of the blood vessels and the other carries the sensation of pain to the brain. Indeed, the only sensation that can be felt within a tooth is pain. The blood vessels, nerves, and branches of the lymphatic system of the body all enter the tooth through tiny holes, called *apical foramina*, at the tip of each tooth root. *(See Figure 2.)*

The root of the tooth, which is generally considered to be that part which is not covered by enamel and is surrounded by bone, is attached to the bone via the *cementum* and the *periodontal fibres*. Cementum is similar to bone and is composed of about 70 per cent *inorganic apatite crystals*, together with an organic element that is largely *collagen* (which is a protein found in many parts of the body). From about the second to the eighth decade of a person's life, the cementum probably trebles in thickness. It receives the principal fibres of the periodontal membrane so that the tooth is secured to the surrounding bone. This important area around the tooth is made use of in orthodontic procedures *(see Chapter 6)* which are involved with moving teeth into more favourable positions under mild pressure. Sometimes, there is a tiny collar of cementum above gum level. If you brush your teeth too vigorously, or if you continually eat a diet which is highly abrasive, this collar can be worn away to expose the exquisitely sensitive dentine.

The *periodontal fibres*, which attach the tooth to the surrounding bone, are between 0.1 and 0.33 millimetre thick. They are constantly stressed by the pressures of chewing, but they are continuously repaired and replaced in a healthy mouth. The periodontal fibres attach the teeth to the bone, to the gum tissue and above the crest of bone, between each tooth, from one tooth to another. The latter being referred to as *transeptal fibres*. Peridontal fibres can be destroyed by the toxins produced by the bacteria which normally inhabit all mouths. Therefore, it is extremely important to control the numbers of these bacteria: if the balance tilts in favour of the bacteria, gum disease and tooth decay will follow.

Thus, the root of the tooth is surrounded by bone and admits nerves and blood vessels into the tooth itself. Therefore, a tooth is not an isolated structure but is very much a part of the body as a whole and the loss of even a single tooth should not be accepted with equanimity. Admittedly, losing one tooth is not so devastating as the loss of a major organ but it is certainly not wise to ignore the fact that the second dentition is irreplaceable and that the first dentition is important in establishing facial growth patterns.

Healthy bone in a healthy mouth is covered by a firm, pink layer of stippled tissue, known as the gum, or gingiva, which is bound down tightly to the underlying bone around the necks of the teeth. Beyond this area, it is more loosely attached and, as it approaches the lip region, it is reflected to form a groove, or *sulcus*. When you brush your teeth, you should begin here so that the entire sulcus, gum, and tooth are cleaned effectively. Perhaps the very name 'toothbrush' has been partly responsible for the prevalence of gum disease, and 'tooth/gumbrush' would give a more accurate idea of the task for which the appliance has been designed. The bone which surrounds each tooth is subject to all the pressures that are transmitted through the teeth which can be considerable. The pressure exerted by a human male's bite between his back teeth is some 25 kilograms per square centimetre (360 pounds per square inch) although it is only about half this figure between the front teeth.

It is also important to bear in mind that teeth only work in pairs; that for each upper tooth, there is also a lower. Therefore, if you lose one tooth its counterpart in the opposing dental arch becomes redundant so far as chewing is concerned. Losing only one tooth alters the bite and this can upset the movements of the jaw and perhaps even cause pain in the jaw joints.

The jaws consist of two bony parts. The lower moveable part is the *mandible* and the upper, fixed part is the *maxilla*. To provide maximum chewing efficiency, the upper and lower teeth should interdigitate with one another when the jaws close, as shown in Figure 3. From a side view, you can best see the situation that is referred to as a normal occlusion (closing). Even the tiniest particle of food can be detected by the teeth when they close together so that you can obviously appreciate the very delicate balance at play during chewing. Recent evidence even suggests that some types of migraine can be caused by an interference in the chewing cycle, associated with the loss of teeth or with the wearing away of artificial or natural tooth substance. These imbalances are detected by the nerve endings in the muscles that are concerned with chewing and the tension that is felt in these muscles can cause considerable stress. Therefore, if you are unlucky enough to suffer from migraine, it would be wise to consult your dentist as well as your doctor.

The jaw joint

The maxilla is fixed while the mandible is capable of a wide range of up-and-down, sideways, and backwards-and-forwards movements. Firstly, the lower jaw adapts to its function of carrying the ten milk teeth, and then the sixteen permanent teeth, during the early years of life by modifications in its shape. This is brought about by reabsorption and deposition of bone at various sites in the jaw bone. One particular area of growth is the *condyle* region of the mandible which provides the articulatory surface of the lower jaw with the temporal bone of the upper facial skeleton. A depression accommodates the condyle, and a disc of cartilage separating condyle from temporal bone divides the joint cavity into

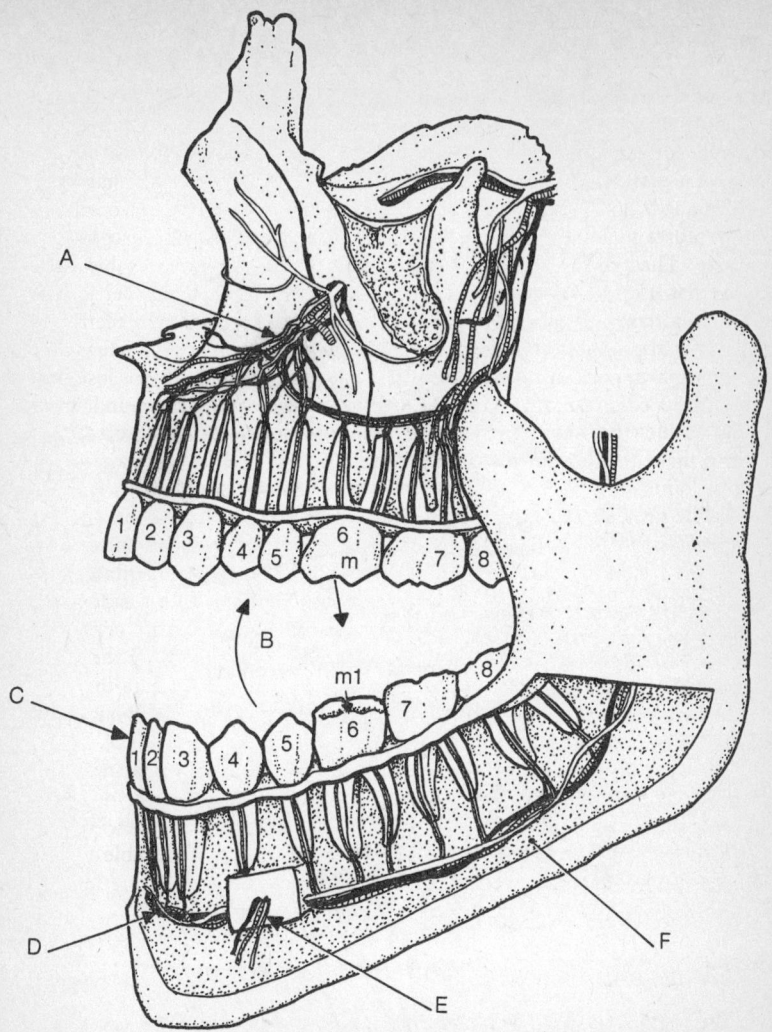

Fig. 3 The occlusion – how the teeth meet. When the jaw closes, the lower teeth close behind the upper front teeth. The upper molar cusp 'm' meets the lower molar at 'm1'. This is referred to as the norm or class I occlusion.

A Blood vessels and nerves supplying the teeth of the upper jaw.
B Shows the direction of closing. m is the cusp of the upper tooth 6 which engages the groove m1 in the lower molar 6.
C The lower incisors touch the backs of upper incisors when jaw is closed.
D Blood vessels and nerves supplying the teeth of the lower jaw.
E Mental nerve supplying the chin region.
F Mandible with bone removed to show the roots of the teeth.

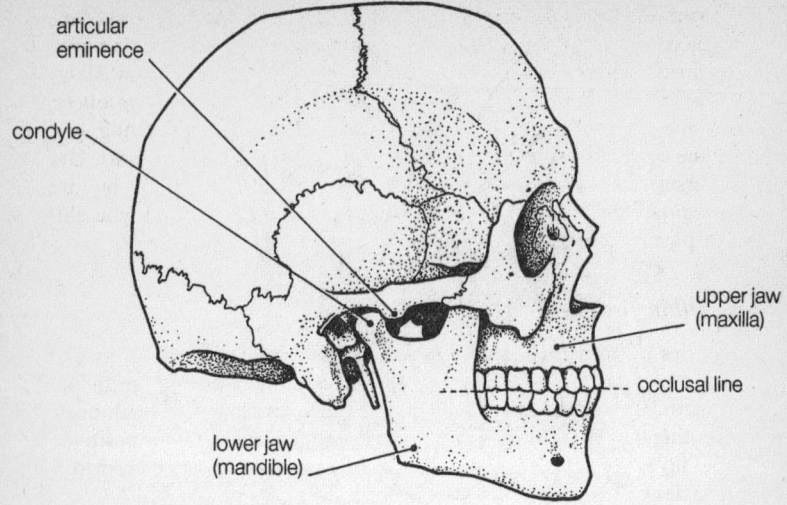

Fig. 4 The skull and lower jaw.

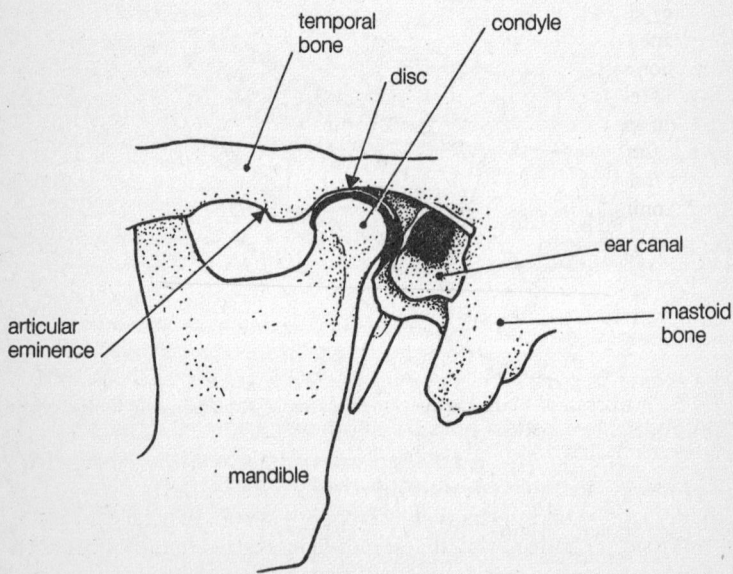

Fig. 4a The jaw joint. (When the condyle goes past the articular eminence an audible click may occur.)

upper and lower compartments. The disc merges into a fibrous capsule which surrounds the whole joint. The condyle can become damaged in arthritis sufferers and, when the capsule itself is less than satisfactory, the condyle can make an audible click as it passes the bony protuberance on the temporal bone. This can be painful as well as annoying and, in some cases, early treatment can be very beneficial *(see Figure 4a)*. Undue pressure can also be brought to bear on the jaw joint by dental irregularities and disease which is yet another reason why you should keep your teeth and gums healthy.

Teething troubles

Stories of sleepless nights for parents and children abound, as do the tales of serious illness associated with the appearance of teeth in the mouth. In fact, we could be forgiven for thinking that our teeth bring us nothing but pain from the cradle to the grave. But, to be positive, we should accept that teething is a perfectly natural event evolved to alter the dentition to adapt from breast feeding, to eating solid foods, and drinking. The process does not come to an end until after the third molars have erupted *(see Chapter 5)* and they, too, may cause discomfort as they appear.

Remember, however, that there is little evidence to suggest that the eruption of teeth causes illness in children. The discomfort that occurs during teething can be relieved by applying certain gels to the sore gums and, in some cases, it may be necessary to give the child a drug to induce sleep. On no account should a drug of this kind be prescribed by anyone other than by a medically or dentally qualified practitioner. It is worth mentioning here that, many years ago, some teething powders contained mercury. Mercury is very poisonous and these powders should never be used. So far as we are aware, such powders have now been banned, but do not be tempted to dig into the old medicine chest for medicines or formulas. When bleary-eyed parents enter a dental surgery begging for help for their teething infants, this is the only advice that can really be offered, except also to suggest that the child is given something to chew on during the day. Once the teeth are through, the real dangers are then from food, drink, and accidental trauma.

Many parents are understandably worried that if their child has some abnormality in the first dentition then the second teeth will be the same. In this case, there is no hard and fast rule, and even the absence of milk teeth does not always mean that teeth will be absent from the permanent dentition. The first teeth are obviously smaller than the second teeth and are usually much lighter in colour. So far as resistance to decay is concerned, there are so many factors involved that it would be impossible to predict whether or not a first tooth is more likely to decay than a second. One thing is certain, however: if a high-sucrose diet is eaten, then there is more likelihood of decay occurring.

If the teeth do not meet or occlude, as shown in Figure 3, treatment may be required to correct the malocclusion as it is called. *(See Chapter 6.)* If the first teeth show any such anomaly, it is rare for orthodontic treatment (a specialized branch of dentistry concerned with straightening teeth in an overcrowded jaw) to be provided. On the other hand, treatment may be given for problems of this kind which occur in the second dentition. Malocclusion in the first dentition does not mean that the permanent teeth will be affected but, similarly, normal occlusion in the milk teeth does not necessarily indicate freedom from the problem in the second teeth.

Sometimes, the malocclusion results from abnormal bone growth such that the upper teeth appear to be very prominent. In other cases, it is the lower jaw which is overgrown and the upper teeth close behind the lower ones instead of the other way round. All these conditions can be alleviated, if not corrected, with expert guidance from orthodontists.

Parents should be seeking advice about dental care for their future offspring while the mother is pregnant. There is insufficient encouragement for the examination of small infants and dentists would be prepared to give sound advice to a pregnant woman. Do not wait until your child has problems before seeking dental advice or think that a particular age is correct to begin dental examinations. The mouth should be examined often to establish the presence or absence of diseases, such as thrush in infants and anaemia in the undernourished. Throughout this book, we shall emphasize that we are concerned with the human body as a whole and not only with the teeth.

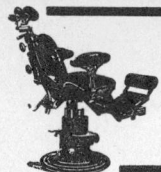

2 TOOTH DECAY, GUM DISEASE, AND THEIR PREVENTION

Almost everyone has seen or felt the effects of tooth decay, but it is surprising how few people are aware of how the disease is caused. *The Guinness Book of Records* mentions tooth decay as one of the most prevalent diseases in the world. There are many factors responsible for the start of the process of tooth decay, as well as many that are responsible for the progression of the disease. We list here some of those factors which have a bearing on it. This list is by no means exhaustive as other things may be discovered in the future.

1 Diet (sugar consumption).
2 Plaque (bacterial activity converting sugars into acid).
3 Tooth resistance – the chemistry of tooth enamel; the shape of teeth.
4 Saliva production.
5 Age.
6 Susceptibility of the sexes to decay.

Like many of our other features, the shape of our teeth is largely inherited and controlled by the genes passed on through our parents. Unfortunately, those of us who have been blessed with teeth that have a pitted or irregular surface are more likely to suffer from tooth decay than those whose teeth are smooth, even, and regular. Normally, the surfaces of the molar teeth at the back of the mouth are more uneven and pitted than those of the front teeth, so that they are the ones which are especially likely to undergo attack *(see Figure 5)*. This is because these areas are more difficult to keep clean and the bacteria that cause decay can lodge here undisturbed for long periods of time. The contact points between adjacent teeth are vulnerable, too, for the same reason. Many people, then, manage to keep their front teeth in good condition for a greater part of their lives while the back ones may be filled with amalgam, crowned, or replaced by a denture.

As you have already seen, the tooth enamel is the outermost protective covering for the tooth and, once again, its make-up differs from person

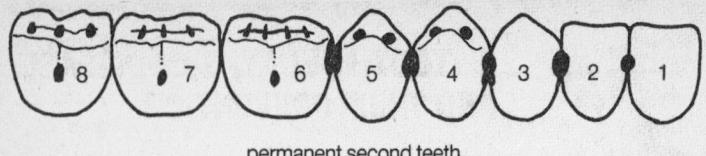

permanent second teeth

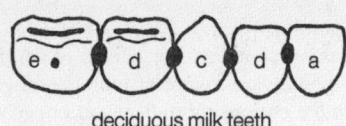

deciduous milk teeth

Fig. 5 The danger areas. All shaded areas are prime sites for bacterial plaque to accumulate and cause decay and gum disease. Compare with photograph 3, in the photo section, which shows a ledgy filling – a further plaque trap.

to person. It is a crystalline material and very tough but the crystal structure of the enamel in one person's teeth may be more resistant to decay than another's. Possibly this may be due to the varying quantities of fluoride in the enamel and, of course, the administration of fluoride has been the subject of much debate for many years. Once again, though, inherited factors may play a part in determining how much fluoride is incorporated into the developing enamel.

Bacteria are microscopic, single-celled living organisms which lack the green pigment chlorophyll and have been described as plants, as animals, or even as some kind of interim stage between. There are many which are harmful and lead to disease while others, such as those that live in the gut of animals including humans, are vital to our very existence. Bacteria reproduce very rapidly so that they can evolve new forms extremely quickly. Indeed, there are even bacteria which feed on the kerosene fuel which aircraft use! Those bacteria that occur naturally in the mouth form colonies on all the surfaces of the teeth and organize themselves on the fine membrane *(pellicle)* that covers every tooth. Together with *mucin*, a sticky component of normal saliva, a coating called plaque is formed. As we have explained, this is more difficult to remove from irregular, pitted teeth.

Plaque is very sticky and it is within the plaque that the process of decay begins. Plaque is a natural deposit but it becomes a problem when

24

a diet rich in sugar is eaten because the bacteria in plaque convert the sugar into acids. This is rather like the process of fermentation whereby yeasts convert sugar into alcohol but, unfortunately, the results are rather less pleasant! The acids that are formed in plaque attack the enamel of the teeth and cause it to dissolve. The bacteria then have access to the dentine of the tooth and eventually to the nerve and blood vessel in the pulp canal.

Sugar is an all-embracing word for a variety of different carbohydrates. The ones that we most often encounter, such as in normal granulated sugar or in many sweet drinks, is sucrose and, unfortunately, this is the main culprit in the initiation of tooth decay, although all sugars should be thought of as potentially damaging to our teeth. The Eskimos of North America provide us with a good living example of the effects of sugar on teeth. Before they began to trade with our culture, Eskimos were relatively free from tooth decay but, over recent years, there has been a dramatic increase in its incidence among these people.

Between the ages of six and twenty-one years, the teeth seem to be most vulnerable whereas, later in life, they are less likely to be attacked and the actual process of decay is slower, too. As one grows older, however, it is more likely that teeth will be lost through gum disease than through decay.

Most dentists are agreed that the presence of fluoride in the chemical structure of a tooth makes it more resistant to acid attack but, during the formation of the teeth, it takes time for the fluoride to be incorporated. Girls' teeth form more quickly than those of boys so that there is less time for fluoride to be taken into the enamel. As a result, they are slightly more vulnerable to decay. Sadly, too, this is enhanced because girls' teeth are more likely to be subjected to sucrose for longer periods than boys' teeth. Sugar consumption is of great importance to the decay process. *It is certainly the frequency with which sugar is eaten rather than the volume consumed which is significant.* The longer sugar is in the mouth, the more time the bacteria have to increase the acid level. Within a few minutes, the acid level increases enough to allow it to begin attacking the enamel. Timing the speed with which acid forms after eating sugar was one of the first important investigations which led to the discovery of how decay takes place.

The first person to carry out these sorts of experiments was R. M. Stephan, so that graphs which show the change in acidity with time after consuming sugar are known as Stephan curves. The graph in Figure 6 plots the pH of the mouth against time in minutes after consuming a 10 per cent glucose solution which is roughly equal to drinking a cup of tea with one spoonful of sugar in it. The pH is a measure of the acidity or alkalinity of a solution and is represented by a series of whole numbers

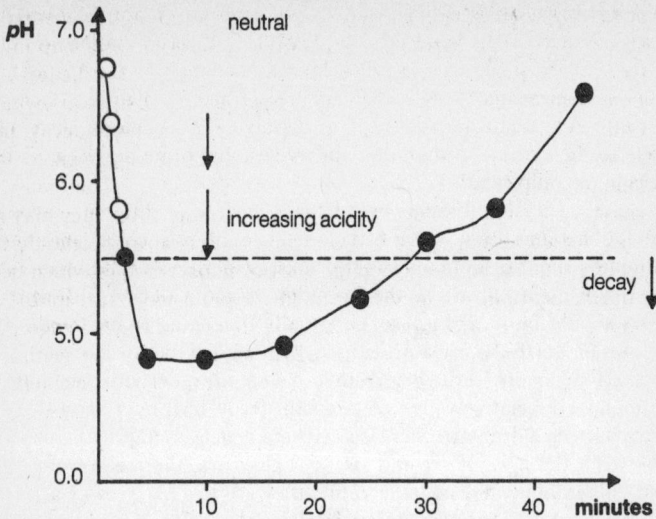

Fig. 6 The Stephan Curve shows the level of acidity in the mouth after ingesting a 10% glucose solution. Note that *p*H below 7.0 indicates an acid solution and at *p*H 5.5 human tooth enamel starts to decay.

from 1 to 14, with the lower numbers denoting increasing acidity and the higher ones greater alkalinity. A neutral solution has a *p*H of 7. You can see from the Stephan curve that drinking a sugary solution causes a marked decrease in the *p*H in the mouth, indicating that the acidity has increased sharply. It is worth remembering, then, that if the *p*H in the mouth falls to 5.5 or less, the concentration of acid is high enough for the enamel of human teeth to begin to dissolve.

It is possible to plot a Stephan curve for any food or drink and, for example, you might be surprised to see the effects after chewing an apple. Although chewing an apple, or other tough foods, does exercise the jaws and stimulates salivary flow, it causes the *p*H in the mouth to fall to as low as 4 which is more than enough acidity to result in the disintegration of the tooth enamel. On the other hand, eating peanuts, cheese, crisps, and, in some experiments, carrots and celery after ingesting a 10 per cent glucose solution, does seem to reduce the acid level of the solutions in the mouth. Chewing tough foods, such as these, leads to an increase in the production of saliva which, among other effects, tends to neutralize the solutions in the mouth. This is referred to as the 'buffering capacity' of saliva and it undoubtedly varies from one person to another. Clearly, therefore, vigorous chewing after a high-sugar diet is beneficial but it will not prevent decay and gum disease altogether because food debris is certain to lodge at the contact points between adjacent teeth. You must remove this debris by flossing. There is one myth concerning the teeth of women which can quickly be dispelled: pregnancy, and the strain which the condition places on the woman's body, do not cause tooth decay, nor is calcium somehow taken from the mother's teeth and given to the developing baby. It is true, though, that some pregnant women may be less careful about diet and, because they may be more tired, they may be more lax in oral hygiene. There is certainly no reason to believe that a mother loses one tooth for each child! The hormonal changes which take place during pregnancy however, do make the gums more susceptible to irritation by plaque. The gums can become quite swollen and engorged with numerous blood vessels which readily rupture when the teeth are brushed. But, when plaque formation is controlled, the problem is greatly diminished.

Gum disease

A dirty splinter in your finger causes inflammation which is indicated by redness of the affected area, heat, swelling, and, of course, pain. Plaque lodged between gum and tooth usually produces much the same effect on the gum. If you remove the splinter, your finger may well bleed as the blood vessels, which have increased in number in response to the irritant, rupture. Similarly, when you brush your teeth and gums so that the previously undisturbed plaque is dislodged, your gums may bleed.

If you were to leave a splinter in your finger for a prolonged period, the infective process may cause more pain, and the battle between the bacteria and the blood's own defence cells results in the formation of yellow pus. Should you remove the splinter at this stage, there may be a considerable flow of pus. In the case of diseased gums, gentle pressure on the area affected by gum disease may cause pus to flow. This used to be called *pyorrhoea* (a flow of pus) but, nowadays, it is more usually referred to as *periodontal disease*, that is, disease of the structures which support the teeth.

While it is hard to tolerate the pain caused by a splinter in the finger for very long, it is rare for diseased gums to be painful. Indeed, one of the reasons why gum disease is so dangerous is because it does not cause pain in its early stages and one is not alert to the disease process which is going on inside the mouth. It is worth remembering that the outcome of gum disease is the loss of teeth when the bone and fibres around each tooth are destroyed. Thus, a completely 'undecayed' tooth can be lost through gum disease. The first sign of this is usually bleeding gums after brushing the teeth. In cases where the teeth are not brushed, which sadly is still a common occurrence, patients are only alerted to the fact that gum disease is present when the teeth are already loose. Therefore, at the first sign of bleeding you must consult a dental surgeon. Better still, don't wait for this to occur, but seek advice from a dentist on how to avoid the problem in the first place. *Gum disease is responsible for a greater loss of teeth in people over the age of twenty-one years than tooth decay!*

Periodontal disease can be stopped once it has begun and a recurrence generally only occurs in the presence of uncontrolled plaque. If you do consult your dentist about 'bleeding gums' your dentist will most likely arrange a programme of oral hygiene instruction for you. This may be carried out by the dentist or by a dental hygienist. Even when gum disease is particularly advanced and the condition is complicated by other problems, referral to specialist 'periodontal surgeons' invariably includes a thorough oral hygiene programme. Many cases of advanced gum disease respond so well to good oral hygiene habits that surgery is rarely performed.

The dentist will resort to surgery when defects in the gum caused by the progress of gum disease actually make it difficult for the patient to remove plaque efficiently. Where the gum has become inflamed and swollen, a space will exist between gum and tooth *(see Figure 7)* and this is referred to as a pocket. The depth of the pocket is a measure of the progression of gum disease. 'Gingivectomy', which means cutting the gum surgically, is the name given to the operation which seeks to eliminate the pockets that harbour plaque and make its removal more difficult. Where a pocket involves only the soft gum tissue, the defects

Fig. 7 A measuring device inserted into a pocket caused by plaque. (Note loss of bone and migration of gum towards the root apex.) The graduations are marked in millimetres on the probe.

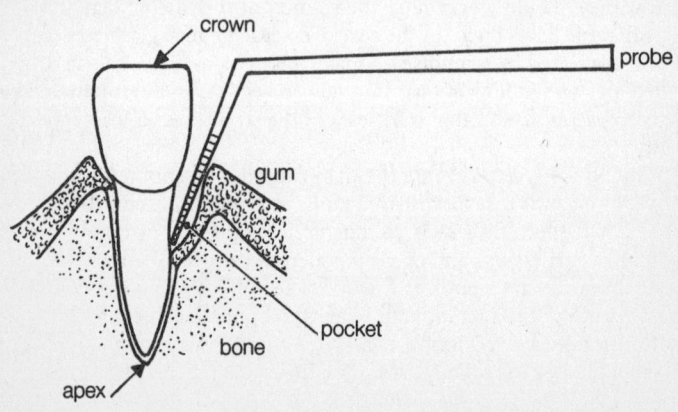

are generally referred to as 'false pockets'. When the disease process has destroyed bone as well as periodontal fibres the defects are referred to as *true* or *bony pockets*. Plaque is the main culprit in the progress of gum disease and, indeed, in its initiation so that it is important to remove any factors which make cleaning the teeth more difficult.

Tartar (calculus) is calcified plaque. It forms to some extent in everyone's mouth but it appears to be more commonly associated with adults than with children. It seems to form more readily on the tongue side of the lower front teeth, and the cheek side of the upper molars. This is not surprising because it is in these regions that the salivary glands open and pour out their secretions. Thus, any plaque in the area will become *calcified* more easily. (This is the process of hardening by deposition of calcium salts from saliva.) Tartar creates yet another ledge on or under which plaque can form so that still more gum disease will result. This is the main reason why a dentist will recommend that calculus should be removed by scaling. A dental hygienist may carry out this important procedure for you, provided that a dentist is present on the premises at the time. Calculus which forms below gum level (subgingival calculus) is often quite unsightly because it gives a dark colour to the overlying gum. Therefore, there is often an improvement in the cosmetic appearance of the teeth and gums after a thorough scaling.

Badly fitting partial dentures, or ledgy fillings which snag dental floss, are also plaque traps. Plaque traps in dentures are unwelcome but, provided that the teeth are cleaned scrupulously and the dentures are not worn during sleep, the dentures are acceptable. Photographs 16, 17, 18, and 19 show the designs for chrome cobalt 'skeleton' type dentures.

Halitosis (bad breath) is not uncommon even in the healthiest person. Sometimes there are obvious reasons for our breath smelling and being offensive to others – smoking and drinking alcohol are two of the best-known causes. Halitosis tends to increase in old age and may be associated with a decrease in the salivary flow, although this has not been conclusively proved. It can be reduced by rinsing the mouth with chlorhexidine mouthwashes, but this should not exceed two short rinses per day because inflammation of the mucous membranes (cheek, tongue, lip, sulcus) can occur, although this is rare. In any event, this should only be carried out in consultation with your general dental practitioner or medical adviser.

Masking the smell of bad breath with mouthwashes should be carried out with caution. A clean, fresh taste in the mouth does not necessarily mean that the mouth is clean and free from disease. Hiding the smell, as it were, is a little like smothering yourself with perfume without bathing.

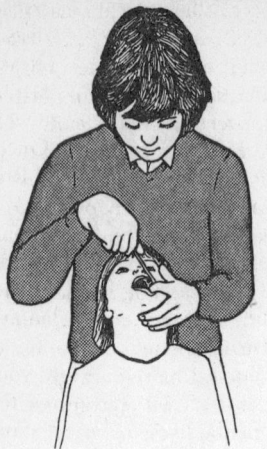 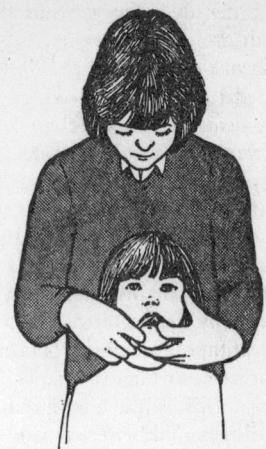

Fig. 8 Positioning for brushing the teeth of a small child. *(Left)* Tip child's head backwards to clean upper teeth. *(Right)* Keep child's head straight to clean lower teeth.

The important thing is to identify the cause of the bad breath. In the absence of digestive problems, lung disease, or even sinusitis, gum disease is a common cause. Thorough mechanical cleaning of the teeth and, in some cases, actually brushing the tongue (without toothpaste) has been known to be beneficial in reducing the strength of the smell. When the problem is caused by gum disease, thorough oral hygiene is the best answer in the long term.

Therefore, because plaque is implicated in the progression of tooth decay and gum disease, it would seem obvious indeed that its very formation should be discouraged. Chlorhexidine mouthwashes do control the formation of plaque to some extent. But, as we have already mentioned, they should not be used to excess, so that we must look towards controlling the amount of plaque that is present in our mouths. Remember that plaque forms in all mouths irrespective of diet, but certain diets do make its effects more damaging, and we shall refer constantly to the main offender, sucrose (sugar).

Plaque is white in colour so that it is not easy to see against the white of the enamel. How many people remark, 'But I clean my teeth; why do I have dental problems?' The reason is simply that many areas of the mouth are not cleaned, even by the most scrupulous. The answer to the problem is to see the plaque. This can quite simply be carried out by staining the plaque with a dye. A simple and relatively inexpensive method is to rinse the mouth with a food dye. Rose pink is one that seems to do the job admirably. There are also several brands of 'disclosing tablets' available, but remember that they are to be chewed to release the dye and not swallowed. It is a good idea to smear the lips with petroleum jelly before using the dyes or you may look as though you are wearing lipstick, although this may not necessarily be a problem. Once the plaque is stained, you can then see it clearly and brush it off. Rinsing alone will not achieve this *(see Figure 10)*.

Disclosing plaque, then, is very valuable for sighted people but the blind cannot use this procedure. Therefore, blind people need careful tuition in oral hygiene measures based on detecting the presence of plaque by the tactile sensations of the tongue, together with an awareness of the stagnation areas which are present in the mouth.

To remove plaque effectively from the surfaces of your teeth, you will need to formulate a plan for brushing methodically each area that is accessible to the toothbrush. The pictures in Figure 9 show a standard method and serve only to illustrate those areas that we consider to be easily accessible to the toothbrush. Your dentist may give you additional advice or, of course, describe a totally different method for you. Every mouth is different and the best method of cleaning is the one which rids your mouth of plaque most efficiently, without damage to the teeth and gums.

Note that some food-colouring dyes contain tartrazine (additive number E102), which is a substance to which some people are allergic. Consult your dentist before using any of the plaque-colouring agents mentioned.

Oral hygiene

There is a bewildering array of toothbrushes on the market these days and it is obviously important to choose the type that is the most effective. In fact, the toothbrush was invented more than 200 years ago, in 1780, by William Addis. It is said that he was involved in the Gordon Riots of the time and that, to escape execution, he hid in a slaughterhouse for horses. It was fashionable then to carve pieces of bone and, because there was also plenty of horsehair in his hiding place, he hit on the idea of inserting the hair into holes in the carved bone and thus he made the first toothbrush. The earliest cleaning aids, however, were probably toothpicks made from twigs, although the Romans certainly fashioned them out of gold. Cleaning the teeth is not the only use to which toothbrushes have been put, and in World War 2 they were made with hollow handles in which maps of Germany, printed on thin paper, could be hidden to assist prisoners of war in their efforts to escape. The first nylon

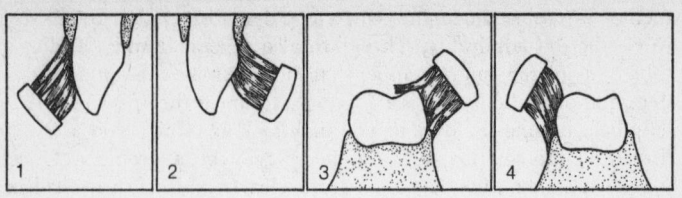

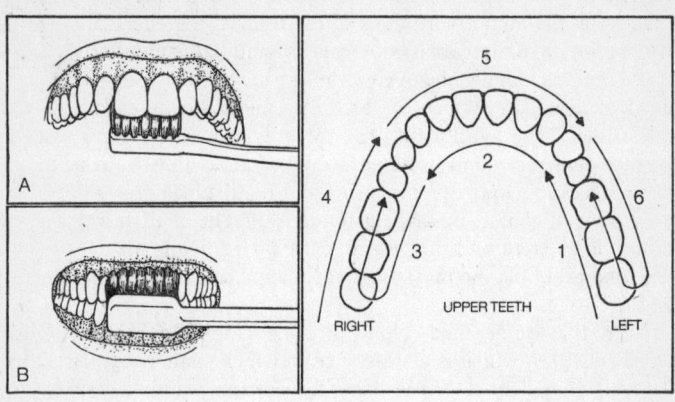

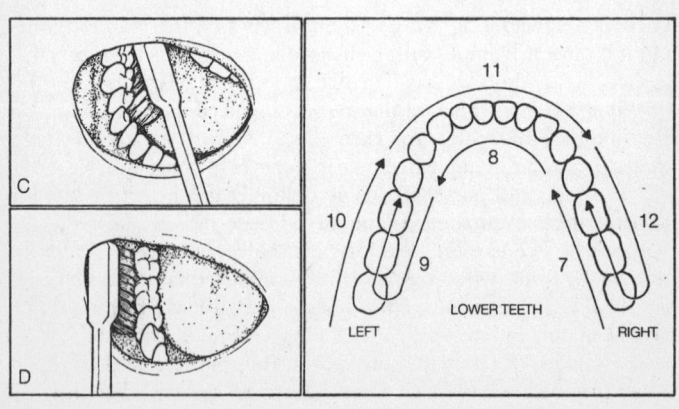

Fig. 9 BRUSH-UP TECHNIQUE. *(Top diagrams)* (Courtesy of Miss A. E. Welham, Product Manager, Johnson and Johnson Dental Care Division, Slough.)

If you brush your teeth in a disciplined manner, effectively, and with the correct toothbrush, your dental health will be improved. 1 Direct the bristles of your toothbrush towards your gum at an angle of about 45 degrees. 2 Use several short, backwards and forwards strokes to loosen particles of food and bacterial plaque from between the teeth and from the small gap between the base of each tooth. 3 Use several longer brush strokes to carry the debris away from the line of the gum and between the teeth towards the biting and chewing surfaces of the teeth. Brush the chewing surfaces thoroughly. 4 Brush gently on the outside and inside surfaces of each tooth, concentrating on just one or two teeth at a time.

THE SECTOR BRUSHING ROUTINE (centre and below). A system for thorough, consistent cleaning.

Diagram A Brushing FRONT teeth – INSIDE surfaces: 1 Start at the *upper left*. 2 Move to *upper centre*. 3 Then to *upper right*. Finish off with the chewing surfaces of the upper right molars.

Diagram B Brushing FRONT teeth – OUTSIDE surfaces: 4 Start at *upper right*. 5 Move to *upper centre*. 6 Then to *upper left*. Finish off with the chewing surfaces of the upper left molars.

Diagram C Brushing BACK teeth – INSIDE surfaces: 7 Switch to lower jaw and start *lower right*. 8 Move to *lower centre*. 9 Then to *lower left*. Finish off with the chewing surfaces of the lower left molars.

Diagram D Brushing BACK teeth – OUTSIDE surfaces: 10 Start at *lower left*. 11 Move to *lower centre*. 12 Then to *lower right*. Finish off with the chewing surfaces of the lower right molars.

toothbrush came on the market in 1937 but, until then, the brush was made from pig bristle.

When you buy a toothbrush, always choose one that has filaments with rounded tips because this type of brush will not abrade your gums. Make sure, too, that the size of the head is correct for you and for your

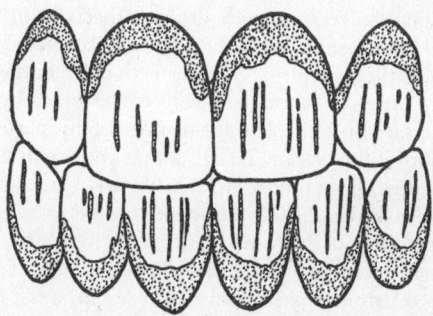

Fig. 10 Plaque displayed (disclosed). Plaque is a white, creamy film which covers the surfaces of the teeth. Under the microscope, it is possible to see the bacteria in the plaque. If you stain the plaque with a harmless food colouring dye, such as rose pink, you will see the plaque on your own teeth.

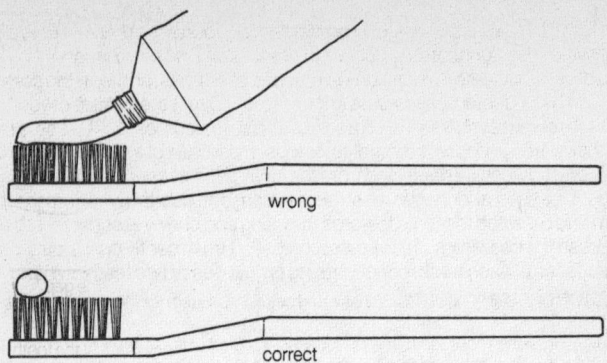

Fig. 11 The correct 'dose' of toothpaste. Don't smother the toothbrush with toothpaste – a small amount is sufficient, about the size of a pea.

children. Some manufacturers mark their products to indicate the size of the head, and the size you need will depend in part on the size of your mouth. Remember that a large toothbrush will not clean your teeth and gums any better than a small one, and you should always be able to use it to reach comfortably into the sulcus and to the back of the last tooth in each arch. It is a good idea to buy a small toothbrush for your child as soon as his or her first tooth appears and, at this time, a baby's natural inclination to put everything in his mouth is a useful one to exploit! Although brushes with natural bristles are still widely available, nylon tufts are much more hygienic, but it is still worth having two brushes so that one can be allowed partly to dry before it is used again.

There seems to be little doubt that using a toothpaste containing fluoride does help to reduce tooth decay, especially in children. Immature enamel does take up some fluoride from the paste and this quite definitely reduces the susceptibility of the teeth to acid attack, although it does not reduce the risk of gum disease. Don't be fooled by the idea that, if you fill your mouth with pleasant-tasting foamy paste with a fresh taste, your mouth is then clean. To check that you are brushing properly use disclosing tablets from time to time *(see Figures 8 and 10)*.

Conventional toothbrushes do not penetrate between the teeth. In a normal adult dentition of thirty-two teeth, there are thirty contact points between adjacent teeth and the surfaces below these points are almost inaccessible to brush and paste and they are only reached by chance. The best way to remove plaque which lodges on these surfaces is to use dental floss *(see Figure 12)* which is a fine thread that can pass easily between the teeth. People commonly complain that floss snags on ledgy fillings between the teeth and that they are frightened of dislodging one.

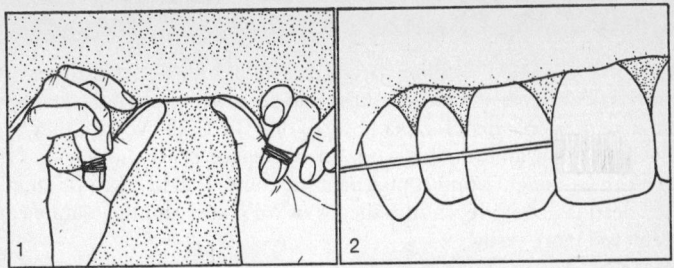

1   Break off about eighteen inches of floss. Wind one end around the middle finger on your left hand and the other end around the middle finger of your right hand. Leave about six inches of floss between the fingers. Pull the floss tight. Place the thumbs and forefingers of both hands on the floss, leaving two inches of floss.

2   Gently slip the floss into the gap between two teeth (one hand has partly to enter the mouth to do this). Concentrating on one edge of the tooth, curve the floss into a C shape around it.

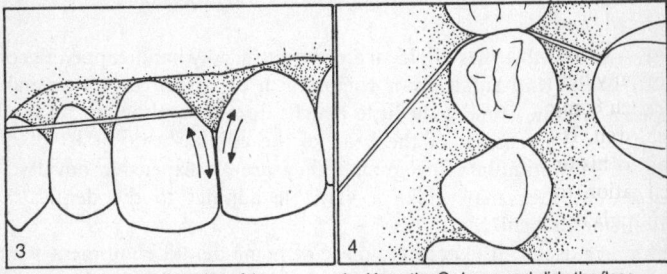

3   Slide the floss up the edge of the tooth to the gum. Gently guide it into the natural space between the gum and the tooth.

4   Keep the C shape and slide the floss back to the biting surface. Carry the floss to the edge of the adjacent tooth and repeat the procedure. Remove the floss from the tooth gap and repeat steps one to three for the other gaps between your teeth, giving special attention to your back teeth. As the floss becomes soiled, wind onto some fresh floss and carry on flossing.

Fig. 12   Flossing your teeth.

In fact, it is useful in itself to discover whether or not you have any ledgy fillings because these should then be replaced by your dentist or, at least, polished using a special strip. If you do find ledgy fillings and these are then smoothed out, you will have reduced the number of potential plaque traps and this aids plaque control. You should also take note if the floss is stained with blood or pus, or if it smells because this is also a sign of gum disease.

Some types of floss are impregnated with a mint flavouring or with fluoride, but remember that the main function of the thread is to remove plaque mechanically. Despite careful brushing and flossing, there are certain areas in some people's mouths that are never cleaned thoroughly. If the mouth is crowded, for example, so that the teeth overlap, they are difficult to clean and, in this case, an interspace brush *(see Figure 13)*, which can be bought at most pharmacists, comes into its own. Its small, tufted head is able to reach into the awkward places and the plaque can be removed more easily.

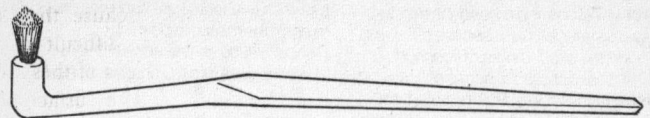

Fig. 13 The interspace brush is useful for cleaning awkward spaces and where there is untreated crowding of the teeth, or around fixed orthodontic appliances.

Electric toothbrushes are ideal aids for physically handicapped people, or for those who suffer from rheumatism or arthritis. A reasonably dextrous person would gain little benefit from one, although no doubt the precise movements of the head of the appliance do assist plaque removal and stimulate the gums. They are an expensive novelty, of course, but they may make a valuable adjunct to the dental care equipment for a child.

Another useful, if expensive, piece of home dental equipment which has recently become available is the 'oral jacuzzi' which can be used for irrigating the mouth and removing particles of debris that lodge in awkward places, such as between the teeth and under fixed bridges, etc. Basically, the instrument is used, perhaps twice a day, to direct a jet of water, at a frequency of about 1,200 cycles per minute, to flush out food debris from between the teeth that may be difficult to remove by brushing and flossing. It is not, however, a substitute for the toothbrush and should never be considered as such. If you use this piece of equipment incorrectly, food debris can be forced into a pocket which may in itself cause an abscess to develop. It is always wise to seek professional advice before using this appliance, especially if you have ever suffered from rheumatic fever or any of the other conditions that we mention in Chapter 8. The jet of water can perhaps cause bacteria to enter the blood vessels around the gum and teeth. On the other hand, there is no evidence to suggest that these high-pressure water devices can cause damage to teeth or to filling materials.

If your teeth have wide spaces between them, the accessible surfaces can be cleaned by using strips of J-cloth about 8–10 cm long and about 1.5 cm wide. The material is quite absorbent and cleans the wider surfaces more easily than a fine strand of dental floss. It is especially useful when teeth have migrated out of their natural position because of the premature loss of other teeth. If the contact points between your adjacent teeth are adequate, then food debris should not shred between the teeth. If, however, you are constantly irritated by this problem then you should seek dental advice.

As we have explained, the teeth most commonly damaged by the decay process are the molars at the back of the mouth. It is an oversimplification to say that these teeth decay because they have uneven surfaces but most would accept that they are difficult to clean properly without correct tuition. To protect the surfaces of these teeth, they can be sealed with a type of plastic coating. The surface of the enamel is etched with a very mild acid which is washed away after it has remained in contact with the teeth for about 30 seconds. A liquid plastic material is then applied to the tooth from a dropper, or sometimes painted on with a fine brush. This is then hardened (polymerized) with a light source (which is often intensified) and the effect is to seal the tiny pits and fissures on the surfaces of the teeth so that they are shielded from the plaque. In this way, a child's first permanent teeth can be protected when they appear, at the age of about six years, followed by a second treatment of the remaining molars at about twelve years of age. The treatment does not shield the areas between the teeth, where decay can also begin, and fluoride gels or rinses may be used in conjunction with this method. Unfortunately, this simple preventive measure is not yet available under UK National Health Service dental care and we can only hope that the situation will change in the near future. It would be fair to point out, however, that the use of fissure sealants is a new procedure and its efficiency must be closely monitored before it is put into practice on a large scale.

Fluoride

It has been proven conclusively, by statistical evidence in the USA, and from a survey carried out in Birmingham, UK, that, if fluoride is added to drinking water, the incidence of dental decay among those who drink the water from an early age really does decrease. The precise way in which the fluoride is effective is not fully understood but it seems likely that the enamel takes up the fluoride and becomes less soluble in acid so that the activity of the plaque bacteria is less damaging. There is some evidence, too, that fluoride reduces the acid-producing capacity of the bacteria. It has even been shown that, in the presence of fluoride and saliva, the tooth enamel actually remineralizes so that tooth decay is arrested.

It is true that the amount of decay that occurs among people of different age groups, who live in areas where the water is fluoridated, varies but this can be explained by the fact that, if fluoride is available during the formation of the teeth, maximum protection is afforded. Fluoride also has a localized effect on the enamel of the teeth. It is this factor which has led to the development of various gels and rinses which can be applied topically to the teeth. The advent of fluoride toothpaste has had a most beneficial effect on the health of our children's teeth. Let us now look at the ways in which fluoride can be administered.

Systemic application

Systemic application is the name given to the ingestion of fluoride from a fluoridated water supply, fluoridated milk, or fluoridated salt.

It cannot be stressed too strongly that there is not a single shred of plausible evidence to link the fluoridation of water at a level lower than one part fluoride per million parts of water with the incidence of cancer. This aspect of water fluoridation has received a good deal of public airing. Both the Royal College of Surgeons and the British Dental Association are quite emphatic on the benefits of water fluoridation at this level and equally emphatic about the absence of risk to those who use the water.

Water fluoridation is, however, a political 'hot potato' and, in a democratic society, a vociferous minority can seem to have as much influence as a silent majority. As a result, the forty-year-old debate about fluoridation continues. At the moment, about one in eleven persons in the United Kingdom receives water from a fluoridated supply. As the water authorities are required to provide wholesome water, it would clearly seem to be advisable to add to the water those substances which have been definitely proven to be beneficial. Fortunately, some water has a natural fluoride component so that the controversy concerning its administration to water supplies has not, at least, deprived some people from the benefits of this substance.

There is an impressive amount of information and scientific evidence which extols the use of milk as a vehicle for fluoride administration. It would appear that, although the fluoride becomes bound to the calcium in the milk, there is still enough available to reduce tooth decay. Fluoridating milk has some other major disadvantages, however. Firstly, it is extremely costly compared to water fluoridation. Secondly, it puts an onus on parents to make sure their children drink such milk. Thirdly, as a 'school milk programme' it will omit all those children under five. Finally, and perhaps equally importantly, not everyone likes milk.

In Hungary and Switzerland salt has been used as a vehicle for fluoridation. The liking for salt is so variable, however, that individual intake is a major problem. The concentration of fluoride in salt is 25 parts per million of fluoride.

Although we have included fluoride tablets and fluoride drops under systemic administration, like fluoridated water, the tablets also have a local effect when chewed. It must be emphasized that the use of fluoride drops or tablets should only be made after careful consultation with your dentist and medical practitioner, and that additional advice should be obtained from the local water board and area health authority (in the United Kingdom). In other countries, you should obviously consult similar organizations and individuals. *Only if there is less than 0.7 parts of fluoride per million of water in the water supply, is it considered safe to administer any supplement*, e.g. tablets or drops.

Please remember that different parts of the UK have different water supplies. Indeed, at times of high water demand or when supplies are switched during times of drought, an individual household can receive water with fluoride levels that vary widely. If you are going away on holiday or sending your children away to school, you should monitor any fluoride supplementation very carefully.

Children over the age of six years should be encouraged to chew the fluoride tablets, and there is some evidence to suggest that, in the presence of a good salivary flow, remineralization of decaying areas can begin. Until very recently, it was considered quite safe to administer fluoride in drop form to babies, just two weeks after birth. As there is now some indication that slight mottling of the enamel of our children's teeth is occurring in some quarters, it would be wise perhaps to limit fluoride supplementation until after the infant is six months old. The administration of fluoride tablets to pregnant mothers does not seem to offer any advantage to the developing child so that it cannot be considered wise to take fluoride systemically during pregnancy.

1 Please remember that there is no such thing as a truly child-proof container. Keep all medicines out of the reach of children.

2 Because it has been proven that some fluoride is good, it does not mean that more fluoride is better. Adhere to the recommended dose. Always seek advice before taking fluoride supplements.

Age	Concentration of fluoride in water (in parts per million)		
	0.3	0.3–0.7	0.7
	Milligrams of fluoride per day		
2 weeks–2 years	0.25	nil	nil
2–4 years	0.50	0.25	nil
4–16 years	1.0	0.5	nil

(2.2 mg sodium fluoride contains 1 mg fluoride ion)

Recommended supplemental fluoride dosage
The dose is measured in milligrams per day according to the concentration of fluoride in the drinking water and the age of the child. As explained in the text, fluoride supplementation before the sixth month is no longer considered to confer any additional benefits to the child. (Reproduced by courtesy of T. B. Dowell and S. Joyston-Bechal from the *British Dental Journal*, 1981, No. 150, pages 273–275.)

Topical application

Avoid using fluoride rinses for children under the age of six years. They are also unnecessary if fluoride tablets are allowed to dissolve in the mouth. Daily rinsing does seem to confer an increased resistance to decay than weekly or fortnightly rinsing but, again, we must emphasize that self-prescription is unwise and you should certainly consult a dental surgeon before embarking on such a course.

The manufacturers of fluoride gels have flavoured their products so that children accept their application more readily. In the light of present knowledge, perhaps this is unwise because a child may well swallow something that tastes pleasantly by reflex action. When the dentist or hygienist applies the gel to teeth, he or she will select a closely fitting tray and apply the gel in that to the surfaces of the teeth. This method can be used for both the upper and the lower jaws and the gel is allowed to remain in contact with the teeth for about four minutes. The idea is that the free fluoride in the gel leaches out and is attracted to the surface enamel imparting an increased resistance to decay. It is likely that, in the presence of saliva, early demineralization of the enamel is halted and remineralization begins. This procedure is not recommended for children under the age of six years whether it is carried out at home or in the surgery.

In 1970 only 5 per cent of the toothpaste sold in the United Kingdom contained additional fluoride. By 1978, the figure had risen to 97 per cent. Young children may swallow quite large amounts of fluoride toothpaste, and some products contain substantial quantities of fluoride.

The recommended amount of toothpaste to be used is about 0.3 gram which is about the size of a small pea *(see Figure 11)*. For children under the age of six years, it is a good idea to supervise the brushing procedure.

Overdosage of fluoride supplements is rare but, if you do ingest too much, then you should seek medical or dental advice straight away. Drinking copious quantities of milk will be beneficial but it may be that you will need a gastric lavage (stomach washout). Once again, keep all medicines out of the reach of children.

Protecting the teeth and gums

The teeth and jaws are often damaged in road traffic accidents and the treatment required for injuries of this kind can be extensive. Consequently, we can only welcome the compulsory wearing of seat belts for the driver and front and back seat passengers of all vehicles, as well as the use of crash helmets for motor cyclists. Indeed, we must be thankful that there has not been an overwhelming opposition to these measures by those people who feel that this is yet another invasion of personal freedom.

It is not only in motor accidents that the teeth and jaws can be injured, and the face should be protected if you partake in a variety of sports. Sadly, this is quite often overlooked. For example, before attending dental school, one of the authors witnessed an operation to remove a person's eye which had been hit by a golf ball. This particular accident was probably unavoidable but it does serve to illustrate how careful we need to be when we indulge in even the most seemingly innocuous pastimes.

It is accepted that boxers should always wear gum shields but very few people would think of wearing them when they take part in other sports, such as cricket, football, rugby, squash, horse riding, or even cycling. As well as damaging the teeth and jaws, the impact of a blow to the chin can be transmitted to the skull and cause concussion. A gum shield has a cushioning effect, it is very cheap to make, and rarely involves more than two visits to the dentist to have one properly made and fitted. They are not available under the UK National Health Service and, although they can be purchased by mail order, they should always be made and fitted by a dental surgeon. They really are well worth the small cost and inconvenience involved.

People who work in certain industries where acidic chemicals are used, such as in the manufacture of batteries or lead/acid accumulators, may also risk dental damage. In most factories there are strict precautions to avoid this, but do remember that acid fumes in the environment can actually dissolve in the saliva so that the mouth's acidity is increased *(see page 26)*. We may wonder if acid rain affects the teeth!

There are other industries, too, in which the environment may affect the teeth and gums. For example, fluoride is contained in bauxite, which is the raw material used in the production of aluminium. Thus, anyone who works in the aluminium industry may be subjected to higher levels of fluoride than is beneficial and, rather than further reducing tooth decay, overdosing with fluoride actually leads to an unsightly mottling of the tooth enamel. If the metal, selenium, is present in teeth to a high level, they are more prone to decay. Consequently, anyone living in areas close to industrial plants which produce these and other hazardous substances are at risk and it is important that the levels of these chemicals in the atmosphere should be carefully monitored.

In addition to ensuring that precautions are taken to reduce the levels of dangerous substances to which workers are exposed, including wearing masks to avoid inhaling toxic chemicals, factories should provide facilities to help people keep their teeth free from attacks from potentially damaging chemicals. In such industries, every worker should be given the opportunity to be able to rinse their mouths frequently and brush their teeth and gums.

Vaccination

It has been reported that active immunization against tooth decay has been successful in rodents and in non-human primates. Now, trials are about to begin on human subjects. The success of the immunization programme is the culmination of years of research and anti-tooth-decay vaccination may one day become available. Research continues, however, for the bacteria and fungi which actively cause gum disease. They have not yet been positively identified and, until they have, immunization against this particularly damaging dental disorder is not possible.

Initial immunity only against dental disease is passed naturally from mother to child from the placenta during pregnancy, and from breast milk.

Together with these natural defences, the boost of a vaccine against dental disease may bring an end to tooth decay. But, the introduction of vaccination, fluoridation, and thorough cleaning of the teeth and gums should not be thought of as an invitation to consume large quantities of sugar. Sugar is also responsible for other ills and a leading nutritionist, Professor John Yudkin, has written a book entitled *Pure White and Deadly* warning against the hazards of eating refined sugar. We should all try to reduce our consumption of sugar in cookies, cakes, ice creams, and sauces.

Diet

In a world in which millions of people are starving while those who are fortunate enough to live in affluent societies have more than enough to eat, it is salutary that the commonest diseases are caused by eating the wrong foods. It has been said that 'you are what you eat' and certainly diet and good health are inseparably associated. Such ills as heart and bowel disease, as well as tooth and gum disease, are caused or, at least, exacerbated by eating incorrectly. There is not a perfect way to eliminate sugar from our diet but the amount we eat and its effects can be minimized with a little thought. We are constantly being bombarded with suggestions about the best kinds of foods to eat to ensure sound teeth in a healthy body but it is as well to remember that new research may modify current advice.

'An apple a day keeps the doctor away.' There may be some truth in this maxim but apples do contain natural acids and, if these are allowed to remain in the mouth, they are potentially damaging to the teeth. On the other hand, simply chewing tough, fibrous foods, such as apples, which exercises the jaws and face muscles as well as promoting the production of saliva, is more beneficial than allowing soft foods to represent the bulk of the diet. Saliva, after all, does have a neutralizing affect on acids. But, although it is impossible to avoid some changes in the acidity of your mouth no matter how carefully you choose your diet, eating apples frequently can no longer be recommended for dental health.

It is very difficult to suggest the 'perfect' diet for everyone, particularly when tastes vary from person to person and when culture and environment dictate what can be eaten. There is, however, one food about which there can be little or no argument and which is freely available to every baby – breast milk. An infant should be breast fed if it is at all possible for it is good for mother and baby alike. The mother benefits from the satisfaction of nursing her own child and, in addition, her body produces a hormone during lactation which causes her uterus to contract so that her body resumes its normal proportions. The baby, of course, receives a natural and correctly balanced diet but also takes in cells from the mother which may in turn affect the type of bacteria present in the infant's mouth. In this way, the mother passes on to her child immunity to infection.

We have already mentioned how well the human nipple is designed to develop the correct sucking action in babies, while certain bottle-fed infants may be at a disadvantage. In any case, a baby's teeth should not be constantly bathed in any kind of milk and babies should be prevented from suckling for prolonged periods. Human milk contains milk sugar (lactose) and this can certainly damage newly erupted teeth so that, if a child is breast fed after the teeth have erupted, their smooth surfaces can decay badly. If the child must be bottle fed, you should not add large amounts of sugar to the feed and, whether the baby is breast or bottle fed, afterwards you should always wipe any teeth that have erupted to remove traces of sugar before the mouth's bacteria can break the sugar down into acid.

Breast milk is, in fact, quite sweet anyway and it seems likely that a taste for sweet foods, associated with the comfort of suckling, leads many adults to eat sweeter foods during times of stress. This may be true during pregnancy, and it is well known that heavy smokers trying to break the habit often resort to sucking peppermints or indulging in other highly sweetened foods. Nowadays, there is definite evidence to suggest that breast feeding is becoming more popular and this is certainly contributing to the reduction in tooth decay among children.

It is interesting to compare the composition of cows' milk and human breast milk:

	Human Milk	Cows' Milk
COMPOSITION		
water/100 ml	87.1	87.3
energy kcal	75	69
TOTAL SOLIDS %		
protein	1.1	3.3
fat	4.5	3.7
lactose (sugar)	6.8	4.8
ash	0.21	0.72
PROTEINS % TOTAL		
casein	40	82
whey protein	60	18
ASH, MAJOR COMPOUNDS		
calcium, mg	340	1250
phosphates, mg	140	960
VITAMINS IN MG PER LITRE		
vitamin A	1898	1025
thiamine	160	440
riboflavine	360	1750
niacin	1470	940
vitamin C, mg	43	11
REACTION	ALKALINE	ACID

(Courtesy of the *American Journal of Clinical Nutrition*, 24 August, 1971, page 971, Gyorgy & Paul.)

In view of the fact that breast feeding is increasing in popularity, mothers should be made aware of the fact that prolonged suckling of infants can cause damage to their teeth. The lactose in the milk can cause damage to the newly erupted teeth. If children are suckled naturally beyond the teething stage there should be thorough cleaning of the teeth both before and afterwards. The infant should also be suckled in a semi-upright position. This would hopefully encourage the flow of milk away from the teeth and therefore swallowed by the infant. Tooth decay actually caused by human breast milk is obviously alarming but it is only prolonged and incorrect feeding which causes this effect. In no way do we wish to discourage breast feeding in favour of bottle feeding. (We are indebted to Dr L. Kotlow for permission to refer to his article in the *American Journal of Dentistry for Children*, May 1977 (pages 192–3).

From the table it is easy to see that there are substantial differences between the two kinds of milk. Human milk contains more lactose than cows' milk and it is perhaps because of this that sucrose is so often added to a feeding bottle. Obviously, too, a growing calf needs a great deal more calcium than a human baby. Whichever way you choose to feed your baby, beware of overfeeding – you may be bringing up a 'bonny' child but it may not be a healthy one.

The first introduction your child will have to sucrose, which may damage its teeth, is in the sugar which is added to dried milk formulas. Therefore, after consulting your doctor, it is a good idea to reduce or even avoid sugar altogether.

Babies should not require extra sugar and, if they do take it, it does them harm rather than good in the long term. Indeed, the liking for sweet foods begins at this time or is at least heightened by the action. Most parents begin to give their baby a mixed feed when it is about six months old and, at this age, the infant does require extra nutriments. Again, however, you might be tempted to feed highly sweetened foods particularly when the child is teething. But do be careful when you are feeding proprietary foods because many of them are sweetened and some contain as much as 39 per cent more sugar than others. During teething the baby can benefit from chewing on a hard rusk, but some of these are also sweetened and should be avoided. Gnawing on rusks probably stimulates the circulation in and around the mouth, and the saliva flow is increased, which will neutralize any acids in the mouth that have been produced by the plaque bacteria. Some rusks contain extra calcium, iron, and vitamins A and D. Don't forget that plaque can form in the mouth of a child who has not been fed at all, so that even the first two teeth can be coated in plaque if care is not taken.

Children are comforted by the sensation of suckling at the breast so that artificial teats or comforters have become popular. It is tempting for the parent to 'improve' the comforting effects of the artificial teat by dipping it in syrupy liquids, particularly when many of the proprietary kinds offer the advantage of extra vitamins. Certainly, the vitamins are valuable but they need not be taken as a sweet, sticky medicine which will result in tooth decay. It is unwise to soak a comforter in any sweet substance. Rosehip syrup seems to be a popular choice for this purpose, particularly as it is a very rich source of vitamin C, but it is much better to provide it as a drink and then clean you child's teeth afterwards.

If you have already begun to reward your child with sweets, it is not easy to stop it suddenly, so it is best never to start the practice. You would be better advised to offer other foods, such as nuts which, although they can be expensive, are quite nourishing. But, if your child has been rewarded in this way, do reduce the amount of sweet snacks and wean him or her on to more savoury things.

When your offspring first goes to school, you clearly have less opportunity to guide his dental hygiene habits but there still remains a good deal that you can do. You should give your child a toothbrush to take to school so that he can brush his teeth after any mid-morning snack or after school lunch. Toothbrushes can be bought in small handy containers and even adults should be able to carry one to use at work. Encourage your child to finish the meal with a drink of fresh water and then to brush his teeth.

It may not be a good idea to eliminate sugar from the diet entirely but do remember that it is the frequency of eating sugar, rather than the amount consumed, which is damaging to the teeth. We should like to see manufacturers marking the dangers of sugar on the containers for their foods in the way that health warnings are printed on cigarette packets. Certain mineral drinks are especially acidic and you should be very wary of when and how much of these that you or your children consume. Carbonated, fruit-flavoured drinks are particularly lethal cocktails to encourage tooth decay. Although fruit and nuts are less likely to cause dental caries than manufactured foods, and their fibrous nature does have slight cleansing effect, eating them in preference to sweets and biscuits is still not sufficient on its own to avoid tooth decay and gum disease.

Even medicines may contain sugar and, if your child requires long-term medication, it is worth discussing the effects of highly sweetened medicines with your doctor. Many medicines can be prescribed in tablet or capsule form but, if your child cannot swallow these easily, and must take a syrup, make sure that his teeth are cleaned immediately afterwards. Mary Poppins' advice should have been 'a spoonful of sugar helps the medicine go down and the teeth rot away'. There is one health education department in Northamptonshire that has produced a poster showing a hand holding a toothbrush and a spoon being filled with medicine conveying the message that 'Taking precautions now may save your teeth later'.

Artificial sweeteners – sugar substitutes

Firstly, it is not as yet considered safe to administer artificial sweeteners to baby foods. 'Xylitol', for instance, has been reported to cause diarrhoea so it is clearly unsafe for small infants – and not too pleasant for the rest of us either! 'Aspartame', which is widely used in the United States and is now available in the United Kingdom, is unsafe if taken by anyone suffering from the disease phenylketonuria.

Any artificial sweetener should therefore be treated with great caution and respect. Obviously, these substances are tested before they are introduced on to the market but constant vigilance is essential to avoid tragedies. Perhaps a safer approach to sugar substitution is gradually to wean yourself off it. There is certainly no need ever to introduce it to your children. Because tea contains a rather rich source of the proven decay fighter, fluoride, it seems ironic that some people saturate each cup with the proven agent of decay, sugar. Leave it out – it's better for your figure, too.

Many baby food manufacturers are now producing feeds which contain less sugar but, still, none at all is better. Rusks are often liberally coated with sugar and, for the present, it is wise to take note of those products which contain the least.

There is probably a future for artificial sweeteners but, because sugar (sucrose) is not a must in our diet, it seems unnecessary for us to pursue the issue further.

Out of interest, however, we have listed here some of the foodstuffs which contain sugar that may surprise you. This information is drawn from the labels on the packaging:

Baked beans
Drinking chocolate
Lemon 'cold relief' powders
Mustard
Salad cream
Canned spaghetti
Tomato ketchup

Vegetarianism

Although we have included this section at the end of our discussion of diet, there is an increasing trend towards vegetarianism, and you should not feel that it takes second place in our consideration of nutrition. We have already discussed eating fibrous natural foods as opposed to manufactured foods so it seems reasonable to mention vegetarian eating at this point.

Some kinds of vegetarian diets do lack some of the B group vitamins and, if you are or wish to be a vegetarian, it is a good idea to discuss your diet with a doctor before embarking upon it. Certainly, chewing tough, fibrous foods stimulates the jaw muscles, the teeth, and the gums but you should not overindulge in this kind of chewing. In one instance, the author did examine a twenty-year-old woman who had complained of sensitivity in several of her teeth. The only explanation that seemed plausible was that the enamel of her teeth was very thin in the first place and that changing to a vegetarian diet had worn it away in several places over a number of years. Whatever you choose to eat, moderation is the best policy.

The value of bread

Bread contains neither fat nor sugar and both brown and white bread provides about 15 per cent of the average daily requirement of energy in the form of starch, as well as protein, fibre, calcium, iron, thiamin, etc. Thus, it should be recommended as a useful part of the diet. Don't be tempted, though, to smear it liberally with jam or other confections but accompany it with vegetables, cheeses, and fruit.

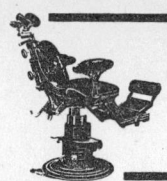

3 TREATING TOOTH DECAY AND GUM DISEASE TODAY

This book is essentially about preventive dentistry. Many people, however, never receive professional dental advice because they are put off by the thought of undergoing dental treatment. We have decided to describe some of the procedures that are carried out to treat dental disease in the hope that with this knowledge 'a visit to the dentist' will seem much less daunting. But there is another good reason for adopting a preventive approach – it is somewhat futile for any repair work to have to be repeated. But, once your mouth has been restored to sound health, you can then begin, with renewed vigour, to develop a high level of oral hygiene. Of course, after the treatment has finished, the well-contoured restorations (fillings and crowns) should make it much easier for you to clean your teeth and gums thoroughly.

The dental examination

There are two sides to a first visit to a dentist – the patient's side and the dentist's side. *(See Table 2 on page 137.)* You should try to explain to your dentist, as clearly as you can, what, if anything, is troubling you at the time, and also provide a coherent summary of your dental history. If you are taking any medication that has been prescribed for you by a doctor or another dentist, it is a good idea to carry with you written details of the treatment. Strictly, it is illegal to treat children under the age of sixteen without the consent of the parents and, although consent is inferred if the child visits the surgery anyway, it is better for a parent to accompany him or her.

When you first visit a dental practice for an examination and/or treatment your dentist will probably begin by asking you a series of questions, or perhaps you will be asked to complete a fairly detailed questionnaire. Try not to be offended by this – your answers are very important and will be treated in the strictest confidence. For example, if you are a woman taking the contraceptive pill, it is essential that your dentist should know because some drugs that are used to treat dental infection may affect the potency of the pill.

You may be asked to provide the following information:

1 Name
2 Address
3 Age
4 Occupation
5 Date of last visit to a dentist
6 Medical history

(This is an extremely important section and the reasons for asking such detailed questions are explained in Chapter 8.)

Tick the conditions (if any) which apply to you.

(a) Have you at any time suffered from rheumatic fever?
(b) Heart disorder of any kind?
(c) Diabetes?
(d) Liver disease?
(e) Disease of the respiratory system, that is, the lung?
(f) Epilepsy?
(g) Have you undergone any major surgery, such as tonsillectomy, in the past?
(h) Do you smoke? If so, how many? Cigarettes, cigars, pipe?
(j) Are you pregnant or a nursing mother?
(k) Do you take any medication regularly prescribed by your doctor or otherwise?
(l) Are you now or have you ever been addicted to drugs of any kind including alcohol?
(m) Have you taken any of the following drugs during the last two years? *(See Chapter 8.)*
     anticoagulants
     steroids *(See Figure 18, p.114*, Steroid Warning Card.)
     tranquillizers
(n) Are you allergic to any drugs?

7 Dental information
(a) Do your teeth or gums cause you pain?
(b) Do you suffer from pain in your jaw joints?
(c) To your knowledge, has any lump or swelling developed around your teeth or jaws?

(d) Have you ever had a tooth extracted?

(e) After a tooth has been extracted or after an injury, do you bleed excessively?

(f) Do any members of your family bleed excessively?

(g) Do your gums bleed when you brush your teeth and gums?

(h) When was the last time a dentist took radiographic pictures of your teeth?

The last question on our questionnaire requires further explanation. Radiographic examination involves the use of X-rays; in the doses used in most dental practices, X-rays are not harmful but, in any case, a strict safety code should be adhered to.

Before you are examined radiographically, the dentist or nurse should place over you a lead-lined apron which should shield the thyroid gland in the neck, the breasts, and the gonad region. In fact, it is only when the beam of X-rays passes through the trunk that it is thought to be essential to wear an apron for routine procedures during a dental examination. X-rays can damage those parts of the body, such as the gonads, which contain rapidly dividing cells. Pregnant women, therefore, should not be examined radiographically if it is at all possible but, if it cannot be avoided, the protective apron must be worn.

The frequency with which radiographic examination should be carried out is still the subject of debate. Within the last couple of years, there have been eminent dentists who have advocated that we should only visit a dentist annually rather than every six months, which is the period normally recommended. However, most people do like the feeling of security which six-monthly appointments give them and, of course, it is much more difficult to remember the dates of appointments if a year passes between visits. In any case, so far as we know, there is certainly no danger in having your teeth examined radiographically every six months and, because dental decay can take place quite quickly, prompt diagnosis can save a good deal of discomfort later on.

Radiographic examination of the teeth and jaws provides a wealth of valuable information. The dentist can determine whether the teeth have become decalcified which, in turn, suggests that tooth decay is present, how deep the decay has penetrated, and how close to the pulp it has reached. The X-ray pictures will also reveal the presence of unerupted teeth in the jaw bones and the angle at which the third molars or 'wisdom teeth' might be lying. Fragmented roots of teeth, too, might be shown up indicating previous attempts to extract teeth. In addition, the presence of extra supernumerary or supplemental teeth might be demonstrated *(see Photo 1)*.

Sometimes, teeth may be congenitally absent and this will be established by radiographic examination. It is also valuable for the dentist to ascertain in this way the number, length, and configuration of the roots before any treatment on the pulps of the teeth is carried out. The dentist can check for any fractures of the jaw bone which may have occurred after an accident or injury, and any fractures of the teeth will be revealed too. The pictures will highlight any bone reabsorption which may have taken place as a result of periodontal disease, and the presence or absence of any cysts or tumours in the jaws will be established by this kind of examination.

Radiographic dental examination has a variety of other uses. For example, it has been used on the remains of Egyptian mummies to determine the state of the dentition, and it is sometimes the only method that can be used to identify the remains of bodies that have been burned beyond recognition after an accident. Indeed, forensic odontology, as it is called, is a fascinating subject.

Once the teeth have been thoroughly examined, it is important to check for any disease in the gums and surrounding structures. As we have explained in the previous chapter, periodontal disease leads to the formation of pockets between the gums and teeth. If the depth of these pockets is greater than 2 millimetres, it suggests that the disease is progressing uncontrolled. The dentist can check for the presence and depth of pockets using a special blunt instrument, called a pocket measuring probe, which is graduated in millimetres and which will slide painlessly between the gum and tooth.

Any lumps or areas of discoloration on the gums might suggest that an abscess is developing on the side of a tooth which is not causing any pain. If such an abscess opens up and bursts, a small tract, called a sinus, will form from the pocket or the root canal to the outer surfaces of the gum. This is a chronic infection and should be treated. Remember that it is not just conditions which hurt that may need to be treated, and any source of infection must be eliminated.

If you have had all your teeth extracted you should still be vigilant about the health of your mouth. We do recommend that anyone, including especially the older man or woman, who wears full dentures should visi. the dentist every six months. Elderly people occasionally suffer from vitamin deficiencies and iron deficiency anaemia; these conditions can easily be detected by a dental surgeon from the colour of the tongue and other tissues in the mouth. This would also tend to bring dentists into a closer association with the aged in the community. But young denture wearers can also benefit from regular dental examinations because the mouth often mirrors the signs of other diseases. It is important to investigate the causes of mouth ulcers or any other lumps that 'don't go away'. If you wear dentures and you are aware of soreness in the corners of you mouth, it may mean that your dentures are worn down and should be replaced.

Treating tooth decay

Sometimes, you may find that your dentist does not treat tooth decay at all. In a child's mouth, for example, it may be kinder and more beneficial simply to ensure freedom from pain and to see that the contact areas between the teeth are self-cleansing. Quite often this results in hardening of the dental tissue in the region so that restoration of the teeth is unnecessary. In some cases, painting the surface of the cavities with fluoride actually encourages hardening of the enamel and dentine.

If you look at the radiograph *(Photo 7)*, you will see that decay is present in the tooth marked. To treat this condition, the dentist will begin by injecting a local anaesthetic solution *(see Chapter 7 for further details of controlling the pain associated with some kinds of dental treatment)* so that the area becomes numb. The undermined tooth enamel and decayed or carious dentine can then be painlessly removed with a dentist's drill. Even when the undermined enamel and dentine have been removed, residual decay can still lodge in the tooth and this must be excavated using various instruments. Then the floors of the cavity are probed to make sure that they are hard and healthy. Tooth cavities are named according to their position on the tooth as shown in *Table 2, page 137.*

If the decay has destroyed wide areas of the tooth, the dentist can fit tiny screws or pins into the dentine which will support the filling material. To make this procedure easier and more effective, a stainless steel band is placed around the tooth; it can be tightened or loosened as

Fig. 14 Fissure sealing may be carried out on molars and premolars in both the first and second dentitions. Note that it provides protection against acids which would otherwise attack the enamel but it does not limit gum disease; nor does it protect any other surfaces apart from those biting (occlusal) surfaces shown.
(Left) Cross section through molar showing deep groove 'fissure'.
(Right) Sealant in 'fissure' protecting against acid from plaque.

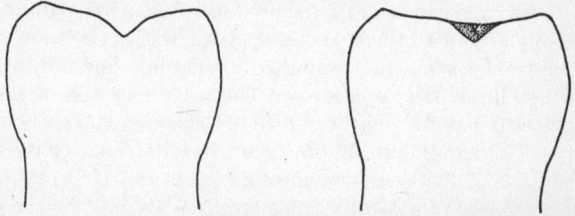

necessary to contour it to the healthy tooth margins. Ideally, the dentist will position small wedges between the band and the adjacent teeth so that self-cleansing areas and surfaces that are easy to clean are provided.

Generally, the cavities are filled with a silvery coloured material called dental amalgam. Essentially, this is a mixture of silver, tin, and mercury, with small amounts of copper added to increase its hardness. Mercury is a poisonous metal, of course but, when it is set, the dental amalgam is harmless and patients are in no danger from it. On the other hand, dental staff could be at risk from mercury vapour which is why the filling material should always be mixed in machines in a well-ventilated area. At first, the amalgam is soft and is placed into the tooth from a special packing gun. Finally, the dentist packs the amalgam tightly against the walls of the tooth cavity.

Fillings in front teeth

Nowadays, these types of filling materials are tooth coloured and are readily available. Originally, white filling materials were a mixture of a form of silica and a mild acid which, when set, was quite resistant to the action of fluids in the mouth. Unfortunately, this material tended to shrink so that, after a while, the filling would fail. It also discoloured. Although the material was the best available for many years, and the acids used were mild, but were inclined to cause some damage to the tooth's pulp, sometimes after many years. Nowadays, a hard, white 'quartz' type of material is used which, while it owes its origins to the original silica compounds, it does not have their disadvantages and keeps its colour-matching properties more effectively.

Like the fissure sealants that we mentioned in Chapter 2, another new technique has now been developed whereby the white filling material can be bonded to teeth. Firstly, the tooth is etched with a mild acid and then the white filling material is bonded to the tooth. Thus, there are no injections, no drilling . . . good news!

Fillings can also be provided in gold, although cost is a limiting factor. In this case an impression is taken of the prepared cavity and a dental technician casts a model from the impression. The model of the cavity is filled with wax and carved to the required shape. The wax pattern is then invested in plaster and, when this has set hard, the wax is boiled out and gold, at very high temperature so that it is liquid, is spun by a casting machine into the hollow in the plaster. The result is a precision casting in gold of the wax pattern which can then be cemented into the tooth. If a large area of a tooth is destroyed by decay, or fractured, or if the tooth is simply unsightly, the whole crown of the tooth can be rebuilt and its appearance will be considerably enhanced. It is not only the film stars of

Hollywood who can benefit from crowns. To make a satisfactory crown is an expensive procedure but clinically acceptable and cosmetically pleasing crowns can be provided at low cost to the patient in the UK under the National Health Service. (*See Photos 8 to 13* in the separate section.)

A cap or crown completely replaces the diseased or discoloured enamel of a tooth but the tooth must be prepared to receive it. Having given the patient a local anaesthetic, the dentist prepares the tooth *(see Photos 8 and 9)*. The thickness of the shoulder around the preparation depends upon the type of crown that is to be fitted and, in Photo 8, we have shown the design for a full porcelain jacket crown. Normally, an impression of the tooth is then made. After root canal treatment has been carried out *(see Figure 15)*, a metal post is inserted into the canal of the tooth and the overall impression taken. When the impression is removed from the patient's mouth, the post comes away with it. From this the dental technician can cast a gold or precious metal post which will fit snugly into the canal. This can then be covered with a porcelain jacket crown. Using this procedure where a post is fitted may be referred to as a 'screw in' type of crown. It is not that the crown is screwed into the bone but that a post is made to fit into the root canal and this is designed to support the artificial crown. *(See Photos 10 and 11.)*

A gold crown can be provided on any tooth from the most obtrusive one at the front to the most hidden back molar. It is a matter of taste. Clinically, however, if the bite is particularly heavy in the molar region, a gold crown is better than one made of porcelain because it has a similar hardness to that of tooth enamel. *(See Photos 12 and 13.)* It is slightly softer than enamel, however, so that a gold crown is less likely to harm opposing teeth. Porcelain, on the other hand, is harder than enamel and may wear away some of the enamel on an opposing tooth. In thin sections, gold is stronger than porcelain, too, so that, in preparing the tooth for a full gold crown, less of the tooth substance needs to be removed. In a porcelain-to-gold bonded tooth, enough of the tooth has to be removed to allow for the thickness of the two materials. Upper molar teeth, which often show when we grin, can be faced with porcelain while the biting surface remains in gold. The colour of the porcelain can, of course, be matched very closely with that of the tooth enamel.

In Chapter 1 we explained why missing teeth need to be replaced. Bridgework restores appearance and function after teeth have been lost and, provided the supporting structures of the teeth are healthy, it is often more desirable to have fixed bridgework rather than a removable denture. For bridgework, a tooth is prepared as if a crown was to be fitted and then the crown is joined to an adjacent tooth so that only the space from which the tooth is missing is restored. Thus, there is no 'plate' in the mouth which can press on the gum and perhaps cause damage. The supporting crowns are cemented to the teeth so that the appliance need not nor, indeed, can it be removed from the mouth. Effectively, it mimics the original dentition and should last for many years. No one need know that you have had bridgework in your mouth and you will avoid the embarrassment that dentures cause among some people. *(See Photos 14 and 15.)*

Root canal treatment

If the decay has reached the pulp of the tooth, it will be painful, sensitive to hot and cold drinks or food, and tender to the touch. The tooth can still be saved by root canal therapy (endodontics). When decay has reached this sorry state, the nerve and blood vessels can be in varying stages of disintegration but, to simplify matters, we shall assume that the decay has only just reached the pulp as shown in Figure 16.

In this case, a radiographic picture of the tooth is taken to reveal how many root canals there are and how long they are. Then, the tooth is locally anaesthetized and access to the canals which contain the nerves is achieved. Next, a fine piece of barbed metal is inserted into the canal to a predetermined length to remove the infected nerve and the canal is dried with paper points. The canal is dressed with an antiseptic solution on a fine paper point and sealed in place with a dressing. If the tooth remains trouble free for a period of about seven days, then a permanent filling can safely be inserted into the canal. There are many of these available, ranging from strips of silver to plastic points. Finally, a permanent filling, inlay, or crown can be placed over the 'root-filled tooth'. Even if the whole of the tooth has been destroyed and the canal has been filled, it is still possible to construct a post crown to restore the tooth.

Abscess

If infected pulp is not treated, the bacteria in the root canal may set up an infection at the tooth's root apex, as shown in Figure 16. This is often extremely painful and requires urgent treatment. In some cases, the infection will spread to involve the glands in the face or neck and there is gross swelling. One way of dealing with this situation is to give the patient a general anaesthetic *(see Chapter 7)* and extract the infected tooth. In this situation it is not always a good idea to use a local anaesthetic because the needle may pass through infected tissue and spread the infection into healthy areas.

In some cases, say, for a front tooth of a young person, the dentist will try to save the tooth. Then the canals can be opened up, as we have

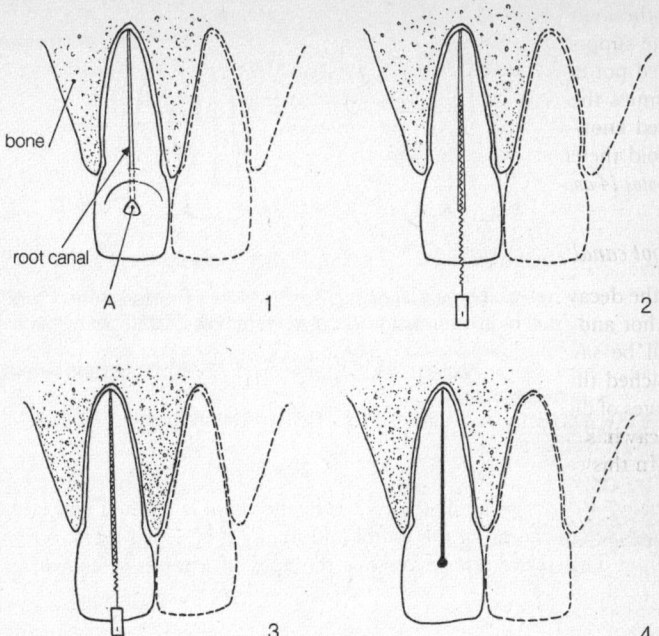

Fig. 15 Root canal treatment. Note that the process is much more complicated for molar teeth with three canals and can be quite time consuming, including several visits to the surgery, if the canals are infected.
1 Hole made in the back of the tooth at A to give access to the pulp in the root canal.
2 Barbed broach used to remove the pulp.
3 Files and reamers used to clean canal. Spiral filler used to spin paste into canal. Gutta percha rods or silver points placed in canals to obtain good apical seal.
4 Gutta percha filling in root canal. Hole in palatal surface filled with amalgam or composite. If the tooth becomes discoloured a post crown can be made. (See photos 5 and 6 in the separate section.)

described earlier, and, sometimes, some of the pus will drain away through the open tooth. If the tooth is treated in this way, the patient will need to be prescribed an antibiotic, such as penicillin, because the infection can continue to spread despite the open canal. If, following this treatment, the area of infection does not diminish in size, the gum over the root can be incised and the bone underlying it removed to expose the apex of the root. This can be cut away and the infected area cleaned with a small, scoop-like instrument. Then the exposed canal is filled with

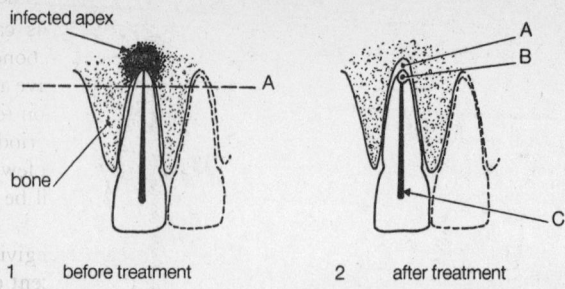

Fig. 16 Chronic infection at the apex of a tooth which has not responded to root canal therapy may require apicectomy, that is, the removal of the apex of the tooth's root.
A Incision line. Gum reflected back. Bone removed. Apex exposed and severed.
A This area infills with bone.
B Cut end of root sealed with amalgam. 'Retrograde amalgam'.
C Root-filled canal.

amalgam *(see page 57)* at the root end, the canal is reamed and cleaned from the crown end of the tooth, and finally it is sealed by an ordinary filling. This procedure to remove the apex of a tooth is known as an apicectomy.

Treating gum disease

If you want to keep your dentition healthy, it is vital to understand the condition of the gum and bone, or *periodontium*, which supports it. This understanding is one of the most important tools in discovering the factors which cause the disease and how it can be prevented. We cannot repeat too often that long-standing gum disease (chronic periodontitis and chronic gingivitis) are the main causes of failure in restorative dentistry. Neither advanced crown and bridge work, nor even simple fillings should ever be provided if the patient suffers from uncontrolled plaque or gum disease. As one dentist summed up the situation, 'It is like putting new windows into a house while it is still burning down!' And, do bear in mind that certain systemic diseases of the body, particularly blood disorders, may increase the susceptibility to gum disease as we have mentioned in more detail in Chapter 8.

It is possible to establish whether or not the patient is suffering from gum disease by making several measurements. The plaque index is a measure of the amount of plaque which is present and is determined by using disclosing solution or tablets. We have already explained how the depth of the pockets between gum and tooth are measured – this is known as the pocket index. If the gums bleed severely, this can be estimated, too, to give a bleeding index. Finally, the amount of bone that has been lost as a result of a given disease can be measured to give a bone index. All of these factors are normally taken into consideration to give an overall picture of the progression of the condition. In fact, periodontal disease is very difficult to measure because it can involve only a few teeth and yet be very severe or involve the whole dentition and still be quite mild.

Among people after the ages of four to five years, gingivitis is extremely common. Indeed, research has shown that 90 per cent of the population of Britain suffers from the disease and, in one study on individuals between the ages of seventeen and twenty-two, all of those examined had periodontal disease. In children under the age of fourteen, it seems that there is more periodontal disease among girls than boys. (This may be associated with hormonal changes which occur at puberty making the gums more susceptible to irritation by plaque.) Similarly, hormonal changes which occur during pregnancy also tend to make the gums more susceptible to the disease. After the age of fourteen, however, boys become more likely to contract the disease because, as the textbooks suggest, it would appear that men and boys are less scrupulous in their oral hygiene. On the other hand, after puberty the prevalence of gum disease as well as its severity decrease until the young adult stage is reached when it increases again. Consequently, it is a great pity that the NHS in the UK has introduced charges for anyone over the age of eighteen because this is bound to discourage young people from seeking dental advice.

Today, the treatment of periodontal disease is being centred more and more upon instructing patients in sound oral hygiene measures, and dentists are assisted in this by well-trained dental hygienists. After the initial examination by the dentist, a series of appointments with the hygienist is arranged to measure the extent of gum disease and to eliminate areas of stagnation where plaque can readily accumulate. The patient's teeth are thoroughly scaled and polished and, most importantly, he or she is instructed and shown how to maintain a healthy dentition. In this part of the book, we are concerned with the 'surgical' approach to treating gum disease but, in Chapter 2, we have explained how mechanical and chemical aids can be used to keep the mouth healthy. Dental surgery should only be resorted to when other methods have not cured the condition completely in conscientious patients.

If the contour of the gums has been altered by the progression of periodontal disease and the condition has not been improved even by good oral hygiene, the gums can be recontoured surgically. This can either be carried out to a limited extent under local anaesthetic or there can be a full mouth recontouring under a general anaesthetic. The purpose of this procedure is to recontour the gums so that all the surfaces can be more easily cleaned. Unfortunately, it is possible that this technique may result in the exposure of the roots so that the teeth appear longer but, if you know that you will retain your teeth, this should be a small price to pay. Recontouring the gum (gingiva) is known as gingivoplasty and is carried out using a high-speed diamond burr in a dental drill or by electrosurgery whereby the gum is cut and the exposed blood vessels heat-sealed at the same time. This treatment is not quite as unpleasant as it sounds but it is still a better bet to control the plaque.

Scaling the teeth thoroughly is perhaps the most important task that can be carried out for you by a dentist or hygienist but it is tiring for dentist and patient alike. Now, however, the recently developed ultrasonic scaler has taken much of the hard work out of the procedure. This instrument, which is water cooled because of the heat that is generated, uses a curved probe vibrating thousands of times per second to produce a resonance that separates the calculus from the teeth. The principle is similar to that which has recently been developed to break up large stones which form in the kidneys. Indeed, kidney stones have a similar chemical make-up to calculus. The stones are broken down into tiny particles which can be flushed out with the urine, thereby avoiding surgery.

After the teeth have been scaled, they are polished to remove any residual staining. Polishing with fine abrasive strips will also eliminate faulty ledges, known as overhangs, on fillings which would otherwise be plaque traps. In the case of heavy smokers where tar has coated the scale itself, scaling may be needed to remove stains but the teeth must still be polished afterwards. Smokers who resort to tooth powders to remove staining should use them with care because they are very abrasive and, if you need to use them more than once a week, you would do better to give up smoking – for the sake of your general health if not for your teeth!

Evidence does suggest that smoking affects the gums. One particular investigation resulted in the belief that the chemicals in cigarette smoke actually reduced the number and efficiency of the body's white blood cells which are normally active in combating infection. Chemicals in cigarette smoke may bind with red blood cell pigment at the site where oxygen would normally bind. It is generally believed that our red blood cells increase in number to keep the level of oxygen high enough to nourish the body. The body's reaction is therefore to produce more red cells. This has the effect of thickening the blood so that more work is required by the heart muscle to pump blood around the body. This is a strain in itself but, in addition, nicotine also causes the arteries to constrict. The tiny blood vessels in the gum may become blocked and fluid will build up in these parts creating a larger number of areas where infection may become more likely. Obviously, we hope that there will be further investigation of the affects of smoking on the gums. It is also proven that the flow of blood across the placenta is reduced in women who smoke during pregnancy.

Do remember that even the very best-designed dentures are a source of irritation to the gum so, if you wear them, you should continue to be scrupulous in your oral hygiene. This is also true in the case of any appliances that are used to straighten the teeth in orthodontic treatment.

The gum and bone are also irritated by the stress resulting from uneven contact due to malocclusion, high spots on fillings, or the different wear patterns of the dental materials, such as porcelain, amalgam, gold, silicates, composites, and acrylic plastics, that are used. All of these may contribute to the strain which can be transmitted to the periodontium via the teeth. Given the same levels of plaque, the extent of gum disease will be increased in a dentition which has been subjected to more mechanical stress.

Where periodontal disease has involved expanses of bone around the teeth, pockets in the bone can develop. This condition must also be corrected surgically. Careful surgery, again carried out under a local anaesthetic, may arrest the progress of the disease. Generally, the bone does not grow again, though the tooth may tighten in the socket. Existing infection can be eliminated by surgery along with the pocket in which plaque could otherwise accumulate.

Gum recession

Some exposure of roots of the teeth occurs naturally as the teeth wear down and overerupt to expose the roots. The teeth become sensitive but there are various toothpastes available which will help to relieve the discomfort. It is a good idea to smear a small amount of one of these pastes on to the teeth so that there is a reservoir of paste on the gum where it meets the tooth. Do ask your dentist first to recommend a particular product to you. This is best carried out last thing at night because the flow of saliva is reduced during the night and the chemicals in the paste have longer to work on the exposed root surface. Even in a young, healthy, plaque-free mouth the gums may recede, however. The canine teeth are surrounded by large buttresses of bone which stand proud of the bone surrounding the other teeth in the jaws. As the toothbrush sweeps across the jaw, more pressure may be put on this bone than on any other part of the jaw bone so that the gum recedes and the underlying bone is resorbed to expose the root of the tooth. The best way to avoid this is to brush your teeth and gums carefully and avoid using a hard brush which can be quite injurious to the gum.

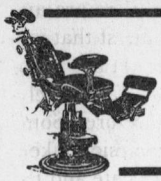

4 DENTURES

In the UK alone, more than eighteen million people wear a denture of some kind, and about two million of these people are under the age of thirty-five. Although it is hard to believe, until recently it was fashionable in some parts of Britain for fathers to arrange for their daughters to have all their teeth extracted and dentures fitted before they were married. The practice was not designed to prevent the daughter from biting her new husband but to save him money and the daughter toothache! Presumably, the thinking was that natural teeth are a nuisance and could be regarded as being expendable. Fortunately today, however, our knowledge is improving and more and more people are keeping a good number of their teeth for longer so that most dentures fitted are the partial ones which replace a few missing teeth rather than a full denture to replace the complete dentition. This does suggest that the preventive dentistry approach is having some effect which is encouraging because, although modern dentures may be cosmetically quite pleasing and comfortable, they are certainly no substitute for the natural teeth. None-the-less, one-third of the population of Britain wears dentures, and even people who wear full sets need to look after their mouths, so we have decided to include a chapter on the making, fitting, and care of dentures.

How dentures are made

Essentially, there are four stages in providing dentures: the impression stage; the bite stage; the try-in stage; and the fitting stage.

The impression stage

After the dentist has examined your gums and jaws thoroughly a impression of your mouth is taken. Impression material which, incidentally, is derived from seaweed, is made up from a powder mixed with water until it takes on a jelly-like consistency. It is then placed in one of a number of standard trays which should conform roughly to the size of your dental arches. If the dentist should then find that there are any discrepancies in the finished impression, he or she may suggest that you return for another one to be taken after the dental technician has made special, close-fitting trays which should fit your mouth more accurately. Indeed, trays of this kind are usually required for partial dentures. Some patients do find one particular difficulty in having an impression taken. Sometimes, the impression material may irritate the soft palate and the back of the tongue which might cause the patient to retch violently. Usually, this problem can be overcome if the patient is advised to relax and breath slowly and deeply through the nose so that, effectively, the back of the throat is sealed as the tongue rises against the soft palate and the vomiting reflex is controlled. In the most extreme cases, however, the dentist may decide to anaesthetize the back of the patient's mouth using an anaesthetic spray.

When the impressions have been taken, they are wrapped in wet tissues and dispatched to a dental technician who pours plaster into the moulds. When the plaster has hardened, the cast is removed from the moulds and covered with a sheet of reddish pink wax from which a wax rim is built up along the dental ridges. These are then returned to the dentist for the bite stage.

The bite stage

This is a vital part of the work and several important measurements must be recorded at this stage. Firstly, the wax blocks are trimmed so that they conform as closely as possible to the dental arch. The distance between the patient's nose and chin is measured with a gauge and the height of the wax is adjusted so that the jaws meet comfortably. The measurement can be based on an existing denture but must account for any wear that will have occurred in the old denture.

Remember that the denture not only replaces the teeth that have been lost but bone as well so that the thickness of the wax in all dimensions is very important because it may often be necessary to plump out the lips or cheeks if there has been much shrinkage or bone reabsorption. The lip lines, too, are drawn on the wax block so that the amount of tooth to be shown can be determined and, at this stage, the centre line of your dentures is also recorded. In consultation with your dentist, now is the time to choose the colour, size, shape, and character of your dentures but you should try to be quite sure of what you want at this stage because, if you want them altered again, it will delay the final fitting of your denture. You may be tempted to match new dentures with your old ones or even look at old photographs of yourself when you had your natural teeth. But take care because dentures should enhance your appearance.

They should be cosmetically pleasing and unobtrusive, and it may be that flashing white pearls showing no signs of wear will not suit your face. After all, it really is not a compliment if a child says to you, 'My goodness, what lovely false teeth you have grandma!'

The try-in stage

By the try-in stage, the technician will have set up the denture according to the dentist's measurements and your personal taste. At this point, any minor alterations to the bite can be made and the appearance of the dentures can be changed if you wish, provided that chewing efficiency is not ignored at the expense of appearance.

The fitting stage

Assuming that all the previous work has been carried out satisfactorily, the fitting stage should be the simplest of all. The dentist will position the dentures in your mouth and check the bite and the appearance. There are various factors, including muscle control, which influence how snugly the denture will fit in your mouth. You will find that the action of your tongue as well as the movements of your lower lip will give some support to the denture as does the upper lip which binds against it. If you have just had old, worn-out dentures replaced, you will probably find that the new ones will feel very large, and any increase in the thickness of the plastic wall will restrict your tongue space a little, as well as altering your speech slightly. Don't worry. This should not last long and may not even occur at all but, even with the best fitting dentures, they may need easing at the fitting stage or later on if they begin to feel tight. After a new denture has been fitted, some patients find that they gain extra confidence by using a denture fixative to hold the new set firmly in place. Many proprietary products are widely available from chemists and you should not feel that you have failed if you use a fixative for the first few days. It should not normally be necessary to use a fixative all the time but your dentist will tell you if it is advisable.

After you have had a denture fitted, you should not feel that you have to live on a diet of soup and soft foods for ever, but it will take a few days, or possibly weeks, before you will be able to master eating hard foods. Dentures will improve your appearance, help with your speech, and make it easier to eat, so it is small wonder that sometimes they do not always match up to the patient's expectations.

Sometimes the dentist may fit an immediate denture as soon as any teeth have been removed. These should not be taken out for at least twenty-four hours after the natural teeth have been extracted because

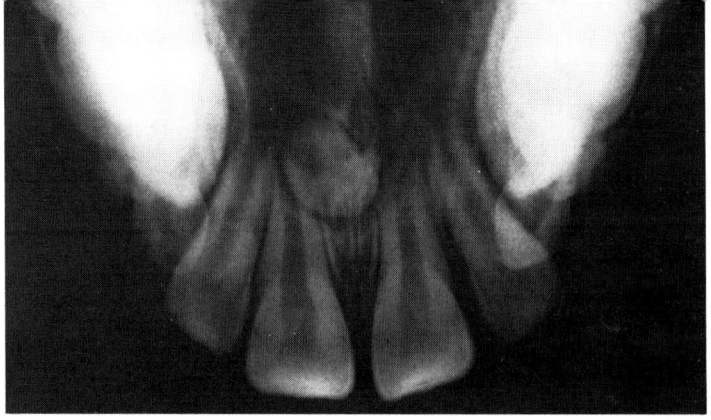

1   A supernumary tooth between two front incisors. The round, white area is the 'extra tooth' which may need to be extracted.

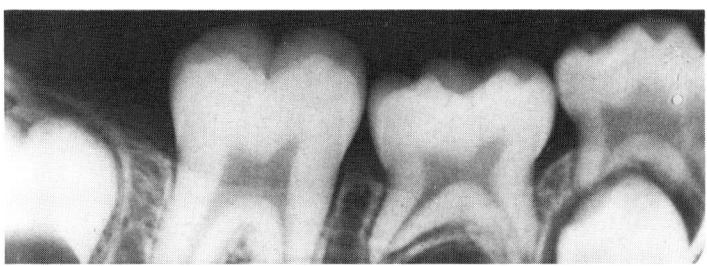

2   An X-ray picture of the lower right side of the jaw of a six-year-old male. Note the second molar forming in the bone.

3   An X-ray picture showing a ledgy filling which will be a plaque trap.

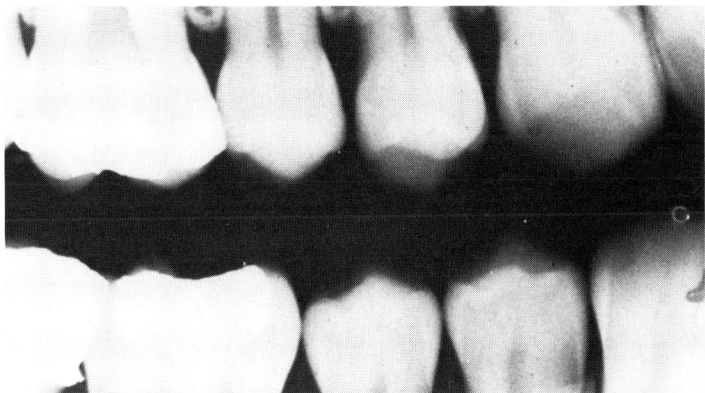

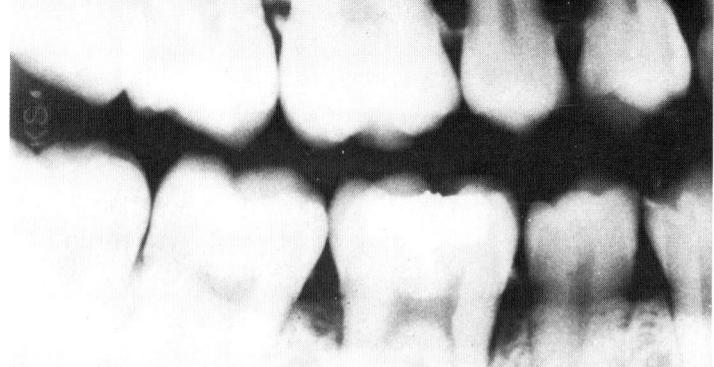

4   An X-ray picture from a thirty-two-year-old male. Note the bone loss around the lower molar and the spurs of calculus attached to the teeth at gum level and below. *(Courtesy of D. A. A. Alexandersen.)*

5   An X-ray picture from a nineteen-year-old female. Note the partially erupted third molar pressing against the second molar.

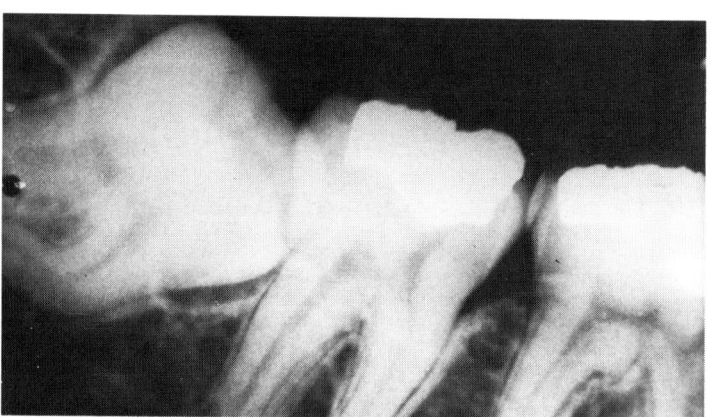

6   Design for dental equipment. This was the winner of the 1973 Melchett Award. *(Courtesy of Richard Satherley, Satherley Design Associates, London.)*

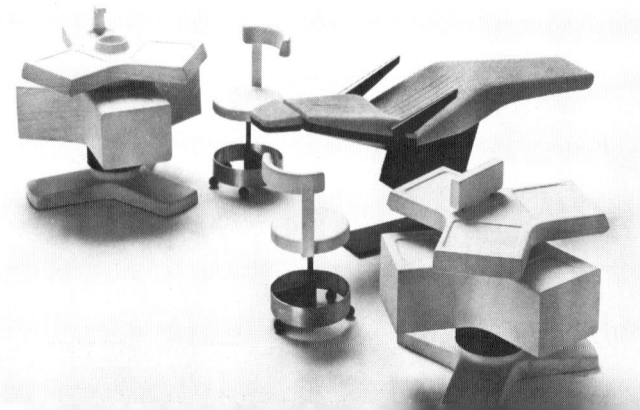

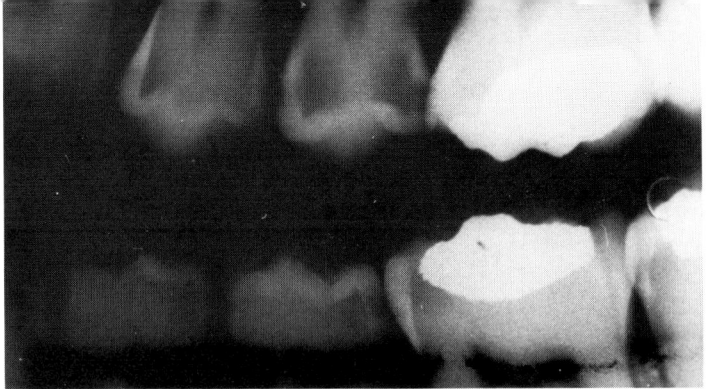

7   An X-ray picture to illustrate decay. Note the dark areas beneath the outer enamel. The heavy white areas are amalgam fillings.

8   A porcelain jacket crown about to be fitted to an upper left central incisor.

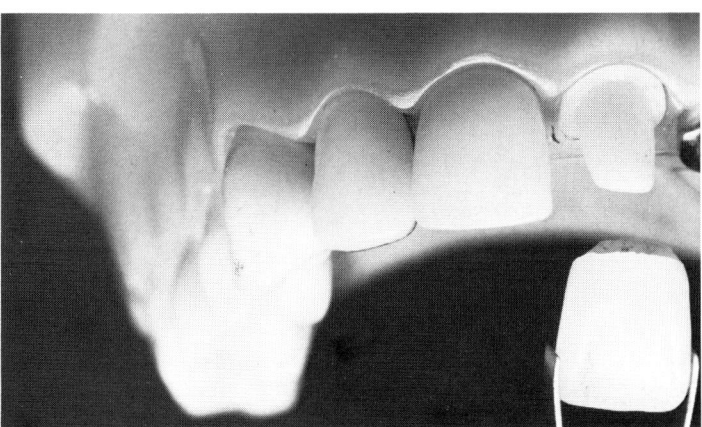

9   A porcelain crown fitted to an upper left central incisor.

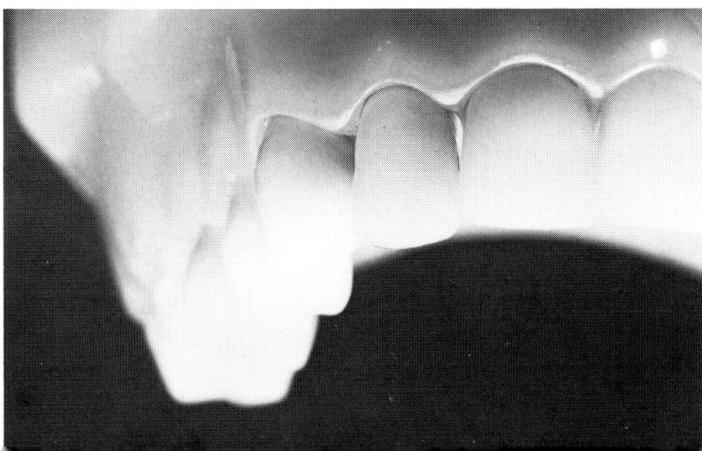

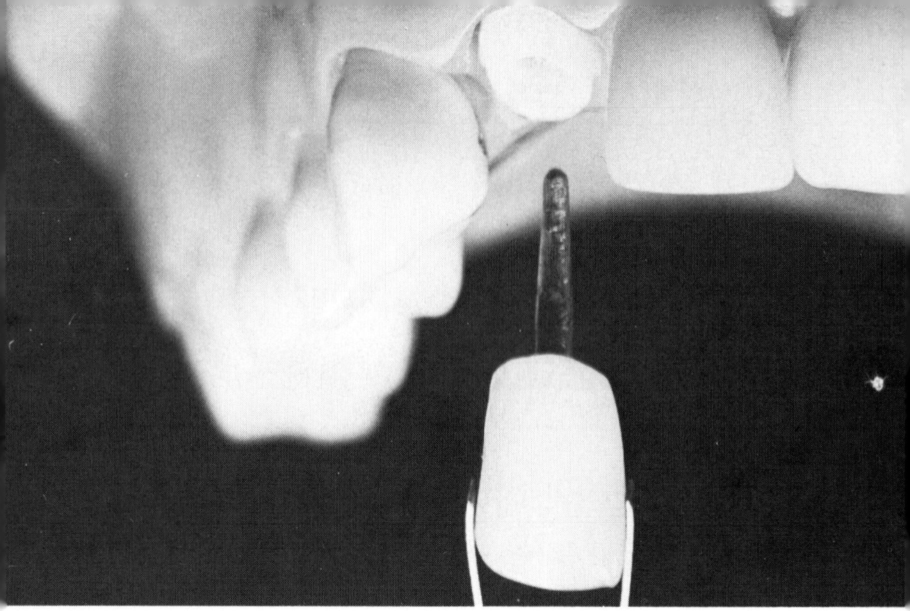

10 A 'screw-in' type of post crown about to be fitted to an upper right lateral incisor. Note that the post goes into the root and not into the gum.

11 A post crown fitted to an upper right lateral incisor.

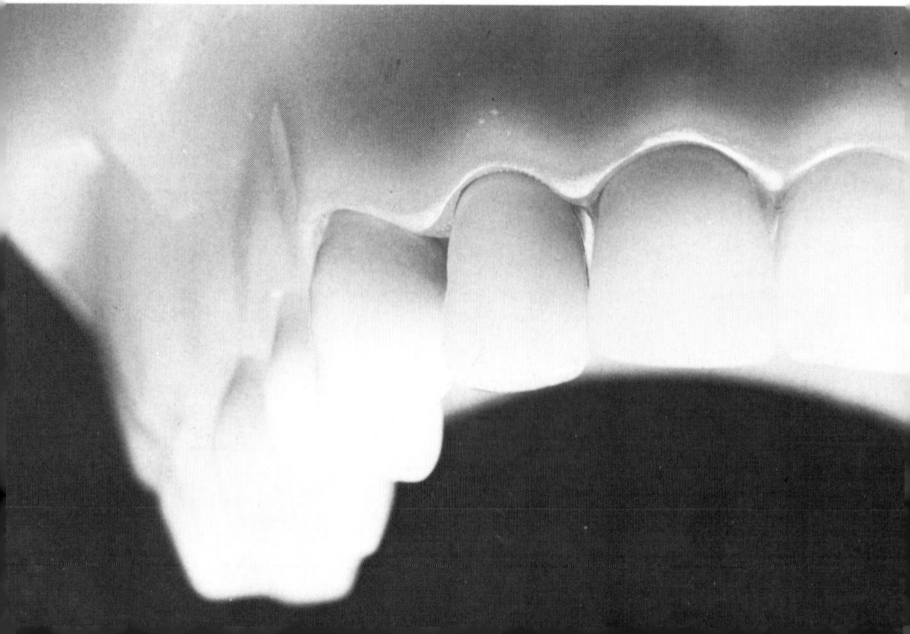

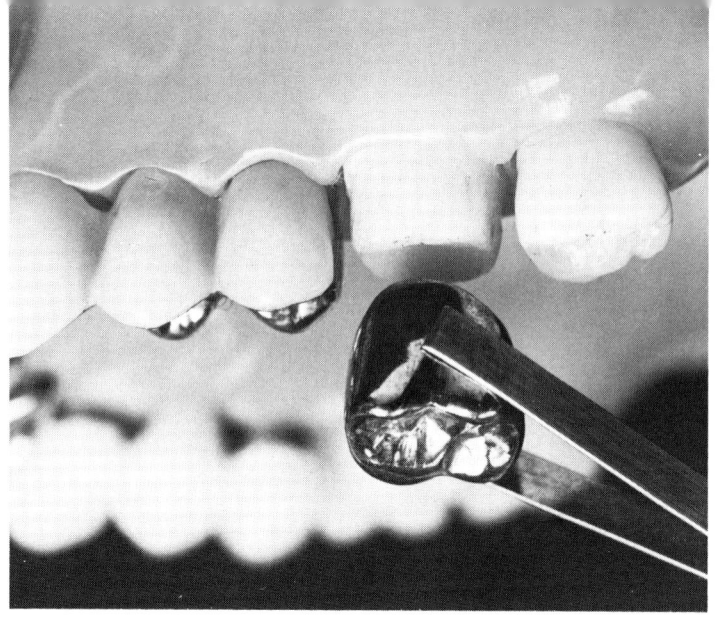

12 A gold crown about to be fitted on to an upper left first molar.

13 A gold crown fitted to an upper left first molar.

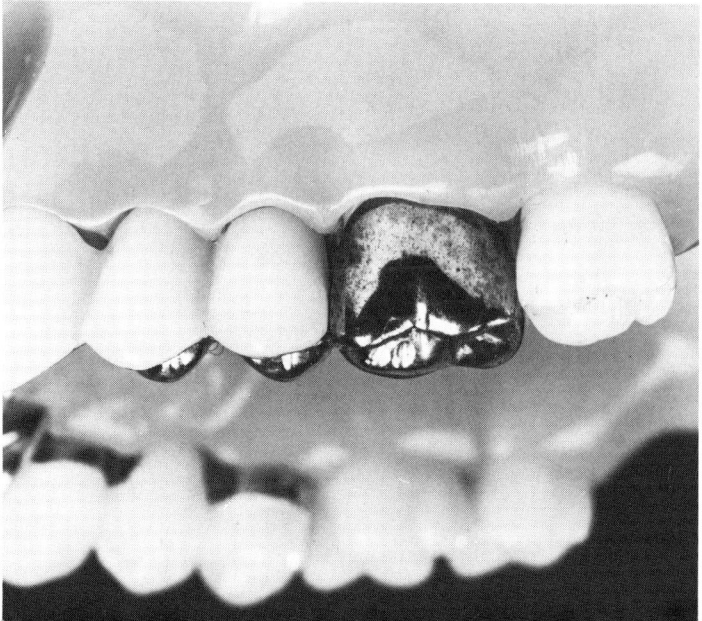

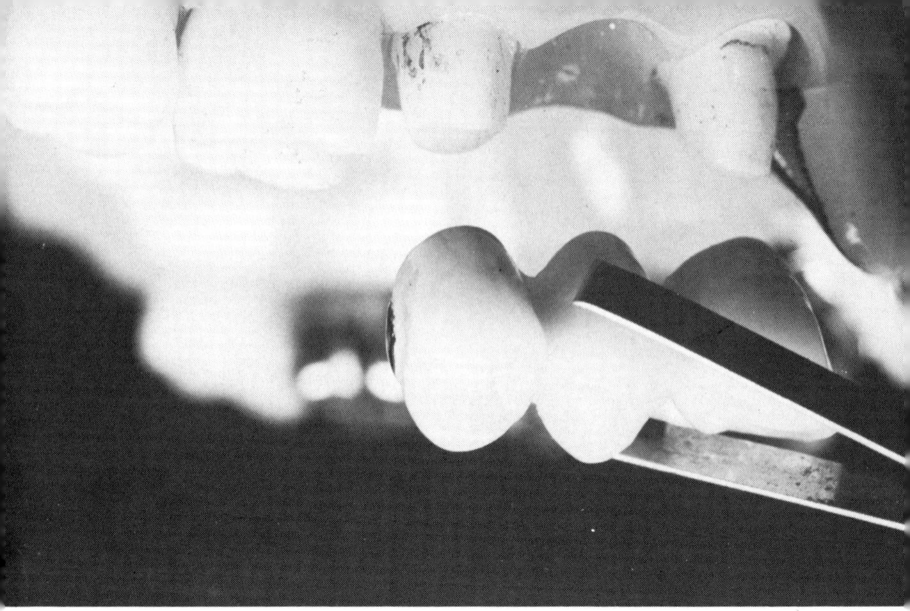

14   Bridgework to replace an upper right first premolar. Note the prepared supporting teeth or abutments.

15   The bridge has been fitted to occupy the space of the original dentition with no plates. Note that the middle unit rests just over the gum. This area must be cleaned by dental floss and/or the use of an irrigation device.

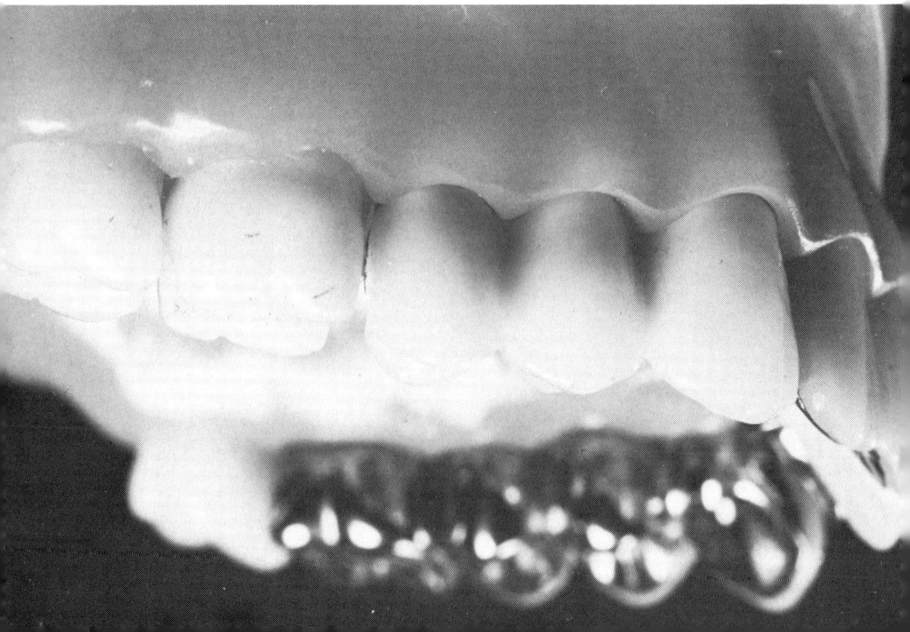

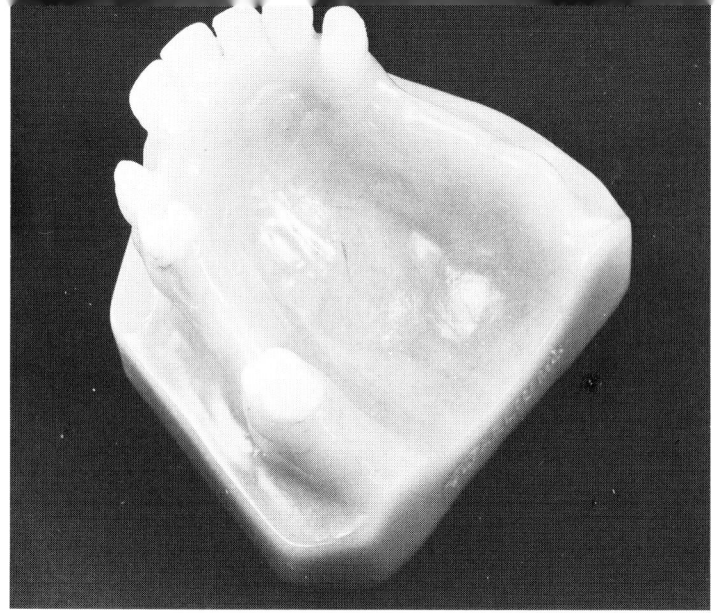

16 A model of a partly edentulous upper jaw.

17 Dentition of the upper jaw restored with a chrome cobalt denture. Note that it is resting on natural tooth and gum and that the palate area is free from pressure.

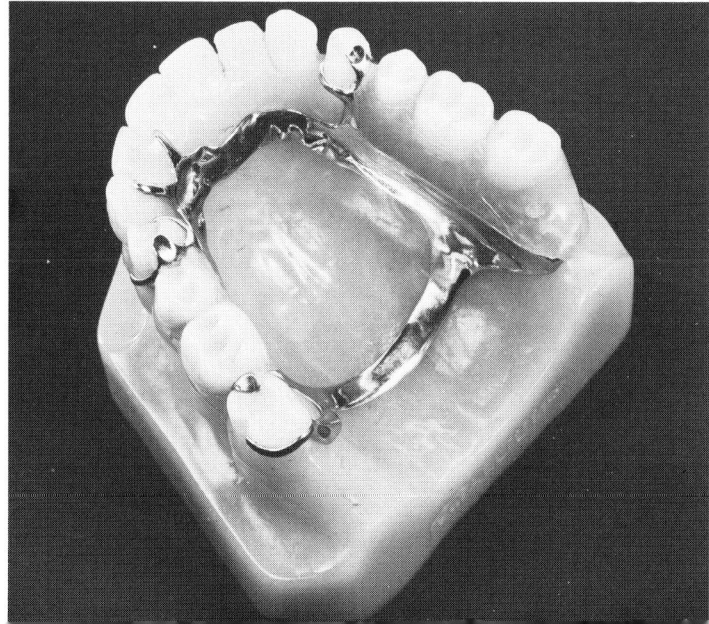

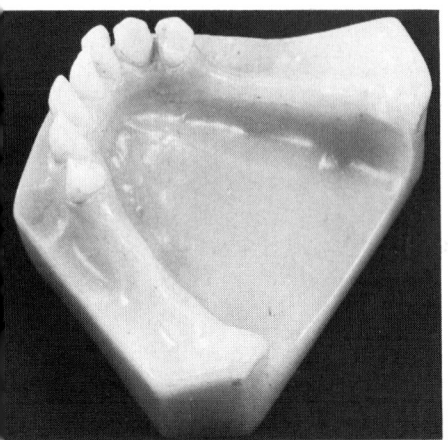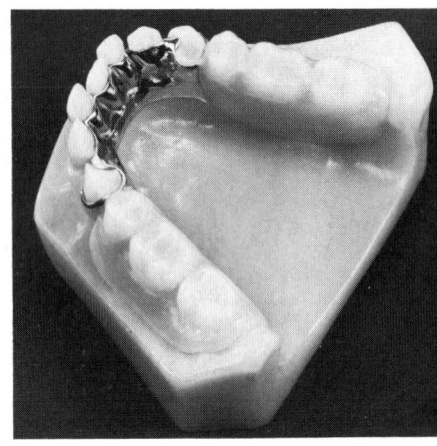

18 *(Above left)* Model of a partly edentulous lower jaw.

19 *(Above right)* Dentition of the lower jaw restored with a chrome cobalt denture.

20 Orthodontic study models. *Top* Class II malocclusion before *(left)* and after *(right)* treatment. *Bottom* Class III malocclusion before *(left)* and after *(right)* treatment. *(Courtesy of Mr Richard Fieldhouse.)*

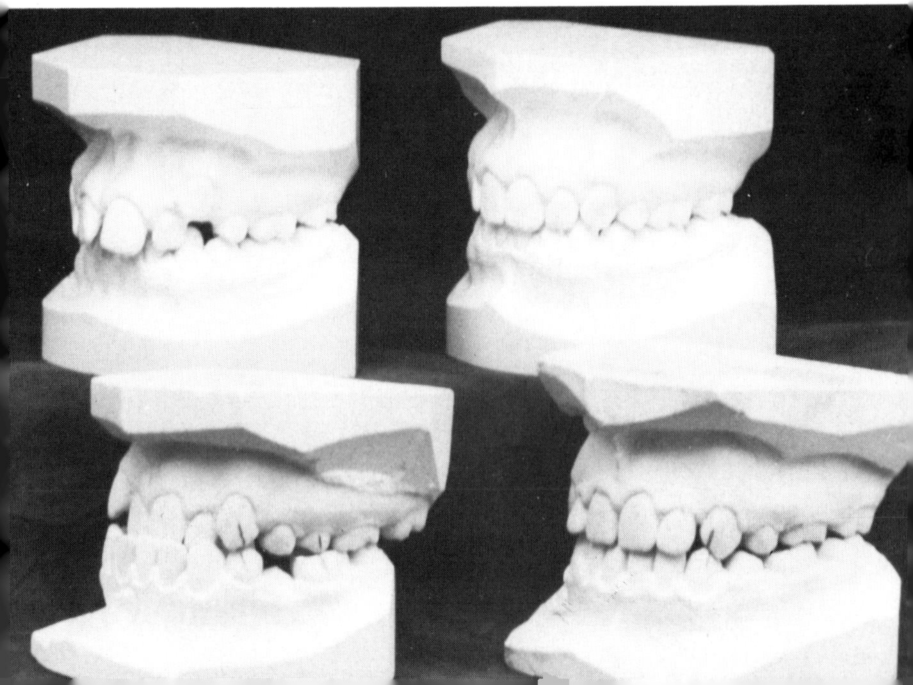

they function as a pack for the bleeding tooth sockets. Initially, therefore, this type of denture should be worn at night. Permanent dentures can also be worn while you are asleep but it is better to remove them because they are 'foreign' to your mouth and the gum tissues do need time to relax. After a few months, immediate dentures may need to be relined because the bone has filled up the sockets from which the teeth have been extracted or has shrunk in other places. This is to be expected and you should return to your dentist to have another impression taken using the denture itself as the impression tray. From this the technician will add more of the plastic material to the fitting surface to improve the fit.

Like your natural dentition, dentures must be kept scrupulously clean. It is a good idea to do this over a plastic bowl filled with water because it is all too easy to drop them on to a porcelain sink or basin when they might be damaged or broken completely. Once again, there are a great many denture cleaning aids available from chemists but it is still worth asking your dentist to advise you. Don't be tempted, though, to use household bleach to clean them, even if they are badly stained, because bleaches will irritate your mouth and craze the plastic of the denture. If they are so stubbornly stained that you cannot clean them with the normal preparations, go back to your dentist; usually, for a minimal charge, he or she will arrange for them to be thoroughly cleaned by the dental technician who will obviously use the correct technique and polishing equipment.

Even if you do break your dentures they can usually be repaired quite quickly – certainly within twenty-four hours. If the work is carried out under the NHS in the UK, it is free of charge at the present but, if the dentist you approach did not fit them, if you require an express service, or if the technician charges more than the standard NHS fee, the dentist may decide that a small charge is required so it is best to ask first.

From time to time, you may find that your dentures feel very uncomfortable. If you think that this has been caused because the design of the denture has mechanically irritated your mouth, it is a good idea to continue wearing the dentures for a few hours before consulting your dentist. This may sound harsh because it will make your mouth sore but, from this, the dentist can easily and accurately locate the site and cause of the problem. It is not just the design of the denture itself which affects how well it fits. If your mouth becomes particularly dry as a result of a decrease in the production of saliva, which may in turn be caused by illness or some forms of medication *(see Chapter 8)*, the denture may become loose. Under normal circumstances, there is a thin film of saliva between the denture and the gum so that the surface tension actually helps to hold the denture in position, rather like the way a thin film of water will hold two flat sheets of glass tightly together. Sometimes, if the mouth is particularly tender, the only solution to the problems of irritation may be to place soft lining in the dentures but, as a rule, these do absorb moisture and are less hygienic than the harder plastic material from which the denture is made.

In some patients, the bony ridges may have shrunken so badly that there is little tissue left to support the dentures, or they may be so irregular that it is inadvisable to fit a denture. In these cases, the problem can be corrected quite easily by minor surgery, often in hospital, to deepen the sulcus and smooth out the ridges. Bearing in mind the huge number of dentures that are provided, there seem to be very few people who need this kind of treatment. If the dentures are very unstable an advanced procedure can be used to implant metal pins into the jaws on which the dentures can rest. Because of the risk of infection around the implants, however, they should be inspected at least every six months, but you and your dentist may decide together that the risks outweigh the possible advantages.

Once again, the most positive approach is to try to conserve the teeth whenever you can. Even though the crown of the tooth has to be lost, it may be possible to save the root. The root can be treated as described in Chapter 3 and then a small stud type of attachment is placed on to the root so that it can be received by the denture to help with stability. The canine teeth, especially, have very large roots which can accommodate

Fig. 17 Overdentures. Note that the cuffs of natural gum around the canine roots must be kept as plaque free as possible.
A   Root-filled teeth (canines) with stud attachment (male) which engages a (female) component in the fitting surface of the denture like a stud fastener.

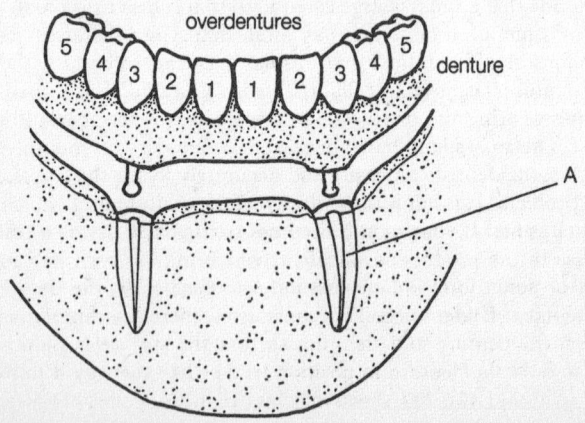

these studs quite readily. This kind of denture is referred to as an overdenture *(see Figure 17)* and, if the teeth are not diseased, they are kept clean, and there is no gum disease, untreated teeth can be covered in this way to enhance the appearance without the need for extractions. It is particularly valuable for teeth that have become discoloured or badly worn down and, because the roots remain in place, there is little or no shrinkage of the bone so that this type of denture is preferable. With prior approval, and if the dentist is willing to carry out the work, this procedure can be carried out under the NHS in the UK but it is a costly exercise. Of course, the supporting teeth roots need to be cleaned very carefully to prevent plaque from accumulating around them. Remember that, just like a dental bridge, the success of a denture depends upon the structures which support it.

Table   Denture materials comparison table

Acrylic plastic	Chrome cobalt	Gold
Cheap to make and a cheap material.	Expensive to make but cheap material.	Expensive to make and very costly raw material.
Weak material – needs to be used in large amounts and cover all the palate.	Very strong material – can be used in fine section. Palate can remain free.	As chrome.
Repairs inexpensive.	Repairs more difficult and more costly.	As chrome.

The table shows the advantages and disadvantages of three commonly used dental materials.

As shown in the table above, partial dentures, which only replace a few missing teeth, can be made from various materials. Whatever material is used, however, good plaque control is essential to the health of the mouth because plaque will attach to the denture itself as well as lodging between gum, tooth, and dentures. Partial dentures constructed from chrome cobalt material have a number of advantages. Unlike plastic, which is not strong enough to be used in thin strips, partial dentures made from chrome cobalt need not cover the roof of the mouth *(see Photos 16, 17, 18 and 19)*. Therefore, although the majority of the taste buds in the mouth are in the tongue, there are a few in the palate and these are left free with chrome cobalt dentures so that eating is more pleasurable. The chrome material is also conductive while plastic has an insulating effect, so that the comforting feeling of taking a warm drink is not impaired by a chrome cobalt denture. Dentures of this kind stain less readily, too, and are easier to clean but, as you might expect, they are more expensive to make than their plastic counterparts.

Gold may sometimes be used in the construction of dentures, particularly if accuracy in casting is important but there is little or no clinical advantage and gold dentures will obviously be costly. Nowadays dentures can be made in virtually unbreakable material although this, too, is expensive. In case of emergencies, some patients ask their dentist to supply them with a spare set. There is no provision for this under the UK National Health Service and it would seem to be something of a luxury which should not be provided by the Welfare State.

Occasionally, it may be difficult to make a partial denture stable in the mouth so that they are made with clasps which fit around the teeth. Patients do complain that these clasps erode the tooth enamel but, if they have been correctly designed, this will not occur and, in nearly every case, it is inadequate plaque control around the clasp which has resulted in tooth decay. Sometimes the clasps are designed so that they rest on as well as around the teeth. This tends to distribute the pressure of the bite to the existing natural teeth as well as to the gum and bone below the denture, so that the denture is said to be 'tooth and tissue borne'. This design is to be recommended because dentures which are tissue borne alone invariably cause undue pressure on the gums resulting in the 'gum stripper' denture.

Very rarely small infants may require dentures because some or all of their teeth are congenitally absent. Anodontia, as it is called, is very alarming for parents who may be comforted to some extent by the knowledge that dentures can be made and that children tolerate them extremely well. Children's dentures must, of course, be replaced very frequently as the child grows. Remember that anodontia may be associated with other illnesses which should be treated by a medical practitioner.

Allergy to denture material has been well documented but, fortunately, it is very rare. If you think that you may have such an allergy, do mention this to your dentist before the denture is made. Then, in conjunction with dental consultants at a hospital, a patch test can be carried out with the assistance of a skin specialist. Samples of denture plastic are applied to your arm and, if a weal develops, it shows that you are allergic to this material. It is unlikely, however, that you are allergic to all denture materials and a compromise can usually be reached.

It has been suggested that full denture wearers should only need to visit their dentist about every five years. We are convinced that this is by no means satisfactory because it assumes that visiting the dentist is only concerned with teeth. But, as we have already explained, the mouth mirrors the health of the whole body and aged people, who are more likely to be wearing full dentures, may suffer undetected vitamin deficiency. This can quickly be diagnosed by the dentist who can then recommend the correct treatment for the patient. Older people are often lonely, too, and welcome the chance to talk to someone, so that their dentist and doctor can be very helpful in this respect. In addition, dentures may wear down and cause soreness at the angles of the mouth – this can be corrected by adjustment. More rarely, it is possible that a tumour can begin in or around the jaws which, because it may be painless, would otherwise remain undetected. If the tumour should be malignant, regular visits to the dentist and prompt treatment may even save life.

As we have explained, the trend today is towards keeping more of our teeth for longer so that full dentures are becoming less necessary than partial ones, but it would still be better if people did not require dentures at all. In any case, we should try to develop the idea that a dentist examines the mouth, jaws, and teeth, rather than just the teeth, and treats the patient rather than just the dentition.

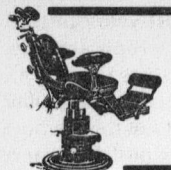

5 EXTRACTIONS, WISDOM TEETH, AND EMERGENCIES

Thankfully, we have come a long way from the time when the tooth drawer would set up his stall in the market place, painfully to remove teeth from the weary poor, which would then be set in dentures for the not-so-weary rich. Despite the progress we have made, however, stories still abound that, 'He had to put his knee on my chest to get the last one out, it bled for weeks, and I'm still not sure he took the right one out anyway!' Don't be put off. Most people like to embellish the facts, especially when it involves the dentist, and tales such as these simply cannot be true today. In the first place, if a tooth does not yield to moderate force (and it was once said that women could not make dentists because they are not strong enough!), then the dentist will take a different approach, perhaps involving minor surgery. Secondly, not even the most robust individual could survive bleeding profusely for more than a few hours without suffering a profound drop in blood pressure. And lastly, although it may be possible for a dentist to extract the wrong tooth, such cases are rare in the extreme.

We continue to stress that you should try to retain your natural teeth and that the best way of doing so is to maintain a strict regime of oral hygiene and visit your dentist regularly. Still, teeth must sometimes be extracted for a variety of reasons:

1 A tooth is causing pain and, despite any proposals for treatment by the dentist, the patient insists that the tooth should be extracted.

2 A tooth may not perform any useful function in the mouth and simply becomes a plaque trap.

3 The tooth has overerupted to such an extent that it fouls the bite and has become hopelessly loose because of its migration out of the supporting bone.

4 The teeth in the jaws are crowded and space must be made so that the teeth can be rearranged orthodontically *(see Chapter 6)*.

5 A tooth has become so loose due to periodontal disease that it is uncomfortable, and any efforts to stabilize it would be unsuccessful.

6 A tooth is buried in the jaw bone and is unlikely to erupt without causing extreme discomfort or will be functionless when it does erupt, for example, an unerupted wisdom tooth in a full denture wearer. *(See photo 5.)*

7 Radiotherapy to treat tumours around the jaws will affect the capacity of the bone to heal so that it may be advisable to extract any suspect teeth before the therapy to avoid any healing problems later.

8 Teeth may be fractured at or below root level in, say, a fight or a road accident. If the fracture is vertical, then it is probably best to remove the tooth. Similarly, if the jaws are fractured, any teeth in the line of the fracture are usually extracted because they may provide a pathway for infection to the healing fracture site.

9 Anyone who is embarking upon a long expedition to a remote part of the world may decide that it is prudent to have suspect or, say, unerupted wisdom teeth extracted to avoid problems or pain while they are away.

10 The patient may decide that there are cosmetic or cultural reasons to have a tooth extracted.

Methods of extraction

It may not always be necessary but, before your dentist extracts a tooth, it may be wise for a radiographic picture of the tooth to be taken to show the angle of the root or roots and the density of bone around the tooth. The picture may also indicate if the tooth has more than the usual quota of roots.

Firstly, of course, the area from which the tooth is to be removed is anaesthetized *(see Chapter 7)*, so having a tooth extracted should not be a painful procedure these days. Then the dentist will use forceps to remove the tooth. There is a variety of types of forceps but they are all designed to grip the root of the tooth, rather than the crown, so there is no need to think you are in for a major ordeal because your tooth is badly decayed or broken down to gum level. In every case, the tips of the forceps are inserted so that their arms press down in the lower jaw or up in the upper jaw, between the bone and the tooth, to sever the attachment of the root to the surrounding bone via the periodontal ligament. At the same time, this also has the effect of expanding the bony socket so that the tooth should yield with only moderate pressure. When the tooth has been removed, the dentist will normally place a gauze pack over the site to reduce the bleeding. It is possible that, after you have left the surgery, this may become dislodged but it is not difficult to replace it yourself and we have included a diagram to help. Almost certainly, your dentist will explain to you any post-operative care that may be required following an extraction. *(See Figure 21.)*

Wisdom teeth

The third molars, or 'wisdom teeth', which erupt after about the eighteenth birthday may cause special problems by becoming 'impacted'. In simple terms, an impacted tooth is one which has not erupted and is either partially or completely embedded in the jaw bone. Usually, it is the impacted lower third molars which are the source of most of the exaggerated stories.

The third molars become impacted simply because there is not enough space in the jaw bones to allow them to erupt. This is partly because there is an evolutionary trend in humans towards a smaller jaw, but also, perhaps, because we eat less tough foods than our prehistoric ancestors,

Fig. 18 Comparison of the jaws of a chimpanzee and a human to show the space available for the third molar ('wisdom') teeth. The ratio of the jaw length to the width of the whole skull is less in the chimpanzee than in the human. The angulation of the ascending part of the mandible is more acute in the human. This may be the reason why there is so often not enough space for the third molars. Other factors are involved but there may be an evolutionary change taking place which is resulting in a smaller jaw in the human while the number and size of teeth remain the same.

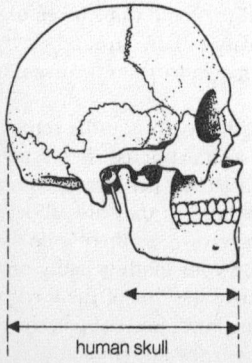

human skull

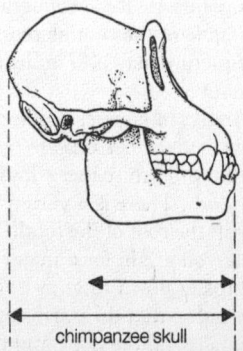

chimpanzee skull

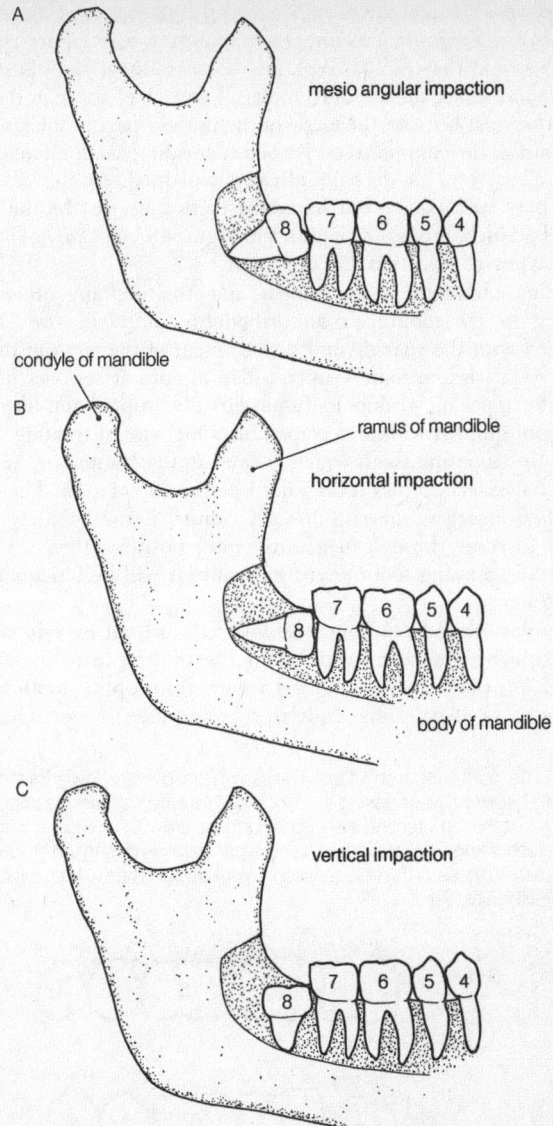

A

mesio angular impaction

condyle of mandible

B

ramus of mandible

horizontal impaction

body of mandible

C

vertical impaction

Fig. 19 The possible positions of impacted third molars ('wisdom teeth') viewed from the lingual (tongue) side. Note that nerves and blood vessels can be very close to the root tips of the third molars.

the apes, which might stimulate growth. If you compare the diagrams of the skull of a chimpanzee and of a human shown in Figure 18 you can clearly see that the chimpanzee's jaw bone is longer than ours so that there is more space for the third molar. The lack of space in the human jaw is worsened because the angle of the upright part of the jaw is more acute than in the chimpanzees. Incorrect suckling as an infant probably has an effect, too, as we have already explained. Any or all of these factors may be involved but impacted teeth may just be the result of genetic bad luck! From the diagrams in Figure 19 you can see some of the various types of impaction that can occur.

Treating impacted wisdom teeth, like treating any other type of crowding in the mouth, is an orthodontic problem *(see Chapter 6)* concerned with the spacing and arrangement of the teeth in the dental arches. As a wisdom tooth erupts, a flap of gum arises over its surface and, if the opposing wisdom tooth has already erupted and bites against this flap of gum, it will be very painful. One way of treating this is to remove the opposing tooth which is causing the trauma or, at least, to smooth its surface so that it does not bite the flap of gum. The erupting tooth then emerges uneventfully. Of course, if the erupting tooth is unlikely to come through in a satisfactory position, then it is best to extract the opposing tooth anyway because it will be functionless. *(See Figure 20.)*

The areas around erupting wisdom teeth are not easy to clean and many problems associated with wisdom teeth are caused by faulty oral hygiene. Any plaque which remains around the erupting tooth can cause the gum to swell painfully. Indeed, it is possible that many problems

Fig. 20 The 'gum sandwich' effect. The flap of gum over the lower third molar (8) is constantly bitten by the opposing third molar. Plaque can also lodge under the flap with the result that an infection is set up around the crown of the lower third molar – this condition is known as pericoronitis. This can happen during the eruption of any tooth, including those of the first dentition. (*Note* Upper 8 has fully erupted. Lower 8 is impacted against 7.)

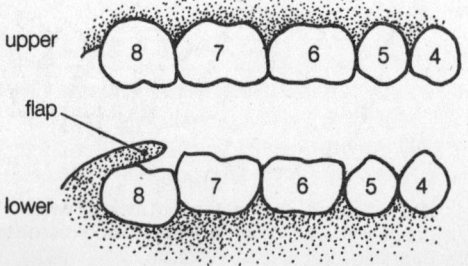

with wisdom teeth are entirely the result of incorrect oral hygiene and you should not assume that because you are the appropriate age and you are feeling pain from the corners of your mouth, that you will have to suffer the discomfort of tooth extraction. Waiting lists for the surgical extraction of wisdom teeth are quite long but your dentist may be able to help you solve the problem simply with advice on dental hygiene.

There are advantages and risks associated with the extraction of problem wisdom teeth and you should discuss the situation with your dentist. The roots of wisdom teeth are close to the nerves and blood vessels which supply the lower jaw. If this is the case, your dentist should mention it to you before any operation is carried out because it may not be possible to avoid disturbing the nerves or even severing them during the extraction. Considering the number of difficult extractions that are carried out, there is only a very small percentage where problems persist but, if the nerves are severed, there is little chance of them rejoining and your lip and tongue may be permanently numbed on one side. If the nerve is only disturbed, rather than severed completely, you will probably feel something like 'pins and needles' and, although it may take many weeks for the normal feeling to return, no permanent damage will have been done.

After you have had a wisdom tooth removed, your dentist will advise you on post-operative care. For every extraction in every individual, the surgery will be different so that only your dental surgeon at the time is equipped to give you the best advice, but we do feel that there are some general points which are worth mentioning.

In all branches of medicine and dentistry, every effort is made to limit the use of drugs and, except for the cases mentioned in Chapter 8, antibiotics are rarely prescribed for routine extractions unless there is an obvious risk of infection. When wisdom teeth are extracted in hospital, however, it is a routine procedure to administer antibiotics to the patient before surgery. You must make sure, therefore, that you do not take any drugs in any form which have not been specifically prescribed for the operation. As we have mentioned before, taking old tablets or other medicines may be dangerous while, if you use only a few antibiotic tablets rather than a complete course, you may risk developing in your body antibiotic-resistant bacteria.

After the operation, you should go home and rest. The dental surgeon will probably give you a pack of gauze to bite on and you should keep it in place over the socket as shown in the diagram (Figure 21) for about thirty minutes. Do not actively rinse out your mouth for at least twenty-four hours because, if you do, you may well dislodge or damage the blood clot in the socket. On the other hand, you can take a luke-warm, non-alcoholic drink after about three hours. If you do

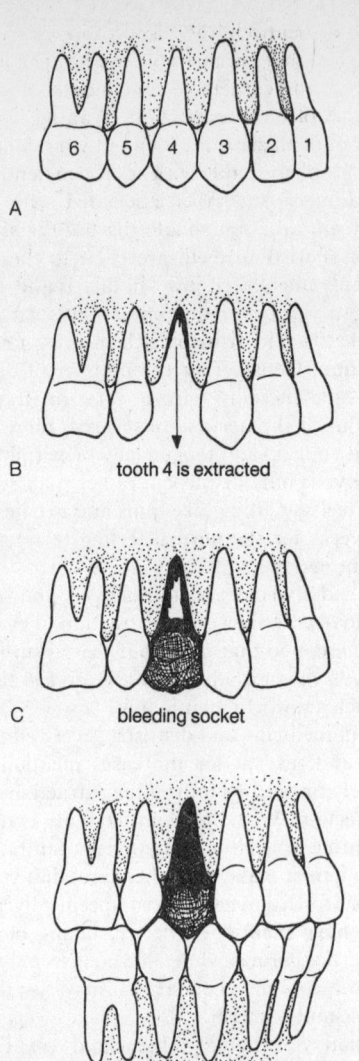

A

B   tooth 4 is extracted

C   bleeding socket

D   gauze pack in place
     patient bites to hold it in place

Fig. 21   The positioning of a gauze pack to arrest the bleeding from a tooth socket after extraction.

dislodge the clot, a dry socket may result and this is extremely painful. This may occur no matter how much care you take. A dry socket may be treated by packing it with a ribbon gauze soaked in a medicinal fluid, and with a prescription of antibiotics. The amount of pain suffered by each individual will vary and the dentist will prescribe pain killers according to need. If you find that pain persists for more than twenty-four hours, to the extent that it prevents you from sleeping, or it interferes with your daily routine, you should seek advice because the pain should not be that severe and may be due to an infection or to bleeding into the tissues. Remember, though, that you have had an operation and your mouth is quite likely to be sore for five days afterwards in the case of a routine extraction, or for as much as two weeks after surgery for an impacted wisdom tooth.

Swelling, known as oedema, is to be expected after surgery but it should not last for more than four days. Interestingly, lean elderly people seem to suffer from oedema less than younger patients. But, it is possible that bleeding into the tissues may occur so that a large blood clot develops resulting in the swelling of the area which becomes painful, and the muscles stiffen. This is treated with antibiotics and the use of hot, salt-water mouthwashes.

When you do rinse your mouth, use a solution of one tablespoonful of salt in a tumblerful of warm water. Avoid any other kinds of proprietary mouthwashes that have not been specifically prescribed because they may contain chemicals which will upset the clotting process. Make sure that the salt solution bathes the area as much as possible by keeping your head tilted on the side of the extraction as you rinse. Don't be afraid to return to your dentist if any condition persists which worries you. Sometimes, you will find that your anxiety will be dispelled simply by the dentist explaining to you what is happening – reassurance is particularly important for children.

Dental emergencies

Bleeding tooth socket

If, after a tooth has been extracted ·or for any other reason, bleeding cannot be controlled, this must be regarded as an emergency. Your dentist will probably have explained to you the action you should take but, in any case, you may find the following advice helpful:

1   A child or an adult should sit down and bite against a clean rolled-up handkerchief or gauze. The pressure of the swab alone may be enough to staunch the bleeding. (See Figure 21.)

2 If after fifteen minutes of this treatment the bleeding still continues, you should telephone your dentist, explain the problem, and arrange an immediate appointment. A child should always be accompanied by an adult. Even an adult should not go alone if he or she is distressed by a bleeding socket.

3 If the dental surgery is closed, then you should try to contact your dentist at home, assuming that he or she is not ex-directory or does not live so far away that it is impractical to see you late at night. In that case, you should get in touch with the casualty department of your local hospital and, nowadays, many counties in Britain run an emergency dental service to cope with just this kind of eventuality. The socket may require stitches (sutures) which does not mean that you have undergone major surgery because sutures are only intended to bring together the ends of a wound so that a healthy blood clot can be retained.

4 An emergency of this kind is best dealt with by a dentist but, as a last resort, you could seek the assistance of your general medical practitioner.

Emergencies in the surgery

Although emergencies are surprisingly rare, it is possible that dental work, which would normally be completely safe when carried out on fit and healthy patients, can cause alarming and perhaps dangerous symptoms if the person is suffering from some ailment which is not obvious. Dentists are, of course, thoroughly trained to deal with emergency situations such as collapse or even respiratory or cardiac arrest. Obviously, it is much better to prevent such a situation and, if you are aware of any illness from which you are suffering or, if you take any kind of drugs, particularly ones such as steroids, anticoagulants, insulin, or antidepressants, you must inform your dentist. In any case, as we have explained in a previous chapter, you will be asked about your medical history on your first visit and it is vital, for your own sake, that you tell the complete truth. If a dentist is in any doubt, he or she will not proceed with the work until a full investigation has been carried out.

Pain is a warning sign and should not be ignored even by the most stoical individuals. Pain in a child may be difficult to track down and, again, you should waste no time in seeking expert attention. Swellings around the teeth, jaws, and face and neck region should also be investigated promptly. If your own dentist is unable to see and treat you on the day that you are suffering, then he or she might be able to arrange for you to see another dentist in the same practice or, indeed, somewhere else.

At weekends and during holiday time, emergency cover is provided in large conurbations. Many local newspapers publish the telephone numbers of duty pharmacists and emergency dental services and, at weekends and during Bank Holidays, local radio stations sometimes broadcast information about emergency dental services. In many counties, local hospitals also hold the telephone numbers of dentists who are involved in the emergency service.

In dental practice emergencies are:

1 Pain.

2 Bleeding from an area where a tooth has been extracted or injury to the mouth has occurred.

3 Acute swelling of the face and neck related to dental infection. This may be associated with an increase in body temperature.

4 Cosmetic problems. In this section, we include difficulties such as breaking your dentures or losing an artificial crown on a front tooth, for example. It is not always likely, however, that a dental mechanic will be available to repair a broken denture and denture wearers should keep one of the denture repair kits to hand, especially during holiday times.

5 Accidental damage to the teeth.

Accidents to the teeth

When a tooth, especially a front one, is knocked out, accidentally or otherwise, then this is a genuine emergency. It is possible that, if you get to a dentist in time, say, within an hour, the tooth can be replaced in the socket successfully. If the tooth has fallen on to a dirty surface, such as a football field, pick it up and wrap it in the cleanest damp cloth that you have to hand. It is always worth making sure that your antitetanus immunizations are up to date and you should be able to tell your dentist if this is the case or not.

If possible, place the tooth in a warm salt-water solution, and arrange a visit to your dentist. Do not remove any strands of gum tissue from the exfoliated tooth. In the meantime, you should bite on a clean swab. When you go to the dentist, take the tooth with you for it may be that it can be replanted in the jaw. The tooth's nerve and blood vessels may already have decomposed by the time you get to the practice and the tooth may need to be root treated before it can be replanted. Don't be alarmed if the replanted tooth turns grey in colour – this is simply caused by the products of blood decomposition in the root canal. It can always be crowned later. Even first teeth can be replanted with the advantage that the spacing of the teeth is maintained. If a small child has a first tooth knocked out so that it literally hangs on a thread of gum tissue, you can place it back in the socket if you are sure there is no risk of the child inhaling the tooth. In fact, in many cases, first teeth retain the integrity of their nerve supply even after a severe trauma because the apices of the roots of these teeth are quite wide and reattach more readily.

A replanted tooth can be stabilized by splinting it to the teeth on either side with a plastic material. Even after a few days the tooth may be quite firm in the socket. Replanting permanent teeth does not always work but there are many instances of exfoliated second teeth being replanted and remaining functional for many years.

Some of the statistics associated with accidents to children's teeth are interesting and worth considering:

1 Even among children of pre-school age, boys suffer more injuries than girls. (Registrar General Reports, 1960. Hardwick & Newman, 1954. J. Dent Research 33.730.)

2 It seems that children from broken homes are more accident prone than those from more stable backgrounds perhaps because any emotional disturbance caused by the break-up of a family may be manifested in violent physical behaviour in the child. (World Health Organisation, 1957. No.118.)

3 Children with protruding teeth in both the first and second dentitions are more likely to injure these teeth than children with non-protruding teeth. In fact, in a survey carried out on a sample of 1,000 children, it was found that teeth are more likely to be damaged in children between the ages of eight and eleven years and that children with protruding teeth are five times more likely to fracture the front teeth than those with normal dentitions. *(See Photos 20, 1 & 2.)* (Hallett, E.M., 1953, Eur. Orth. Soc. 266.)

4 Observations of 118 children at the Turner Dental Hospital in Manchester showed that, among the younger children, trauma to the first teeth was more likely to occur between the ages of one and two years which seems to concur with the way in which toddlers normally behave. (Schreiber C.K., 1959, Br. Dent. J. 106.340.) The roots of

teeth in the second dentition do not become mature until the younger person reaches the mid-teens so that, generally, permanent crowns are not provided for fractured incisor teeth in young people under the age of about sixteen. Temporary basket crowns may be made from white plastic material, however, but the tooth is not prepared so extensively as it would be for a conventional, permanent crown. Even if a crown is not fitted, the young person's appearance can still be enhanced using the acid etching techniques that we have described in Chapter 3.

After a blow to the face, your lips and cheeks may become very bruised and swollen so that your appearance is so distressing to you that you will seek treatment straight away. After a road traffic accident or a serious fall, for example, in which your face, teeth, or jaws have been injured, it is a wise precaution to have a thorough examination in the casualty department of a hospital. This should include a radiographic examination of the skull to check for any other fractures and, only after the doctors are completely satisfied that no other damage has been done, should you go to the dentist. All injuries should be regarded with suspicion until it is proven that all is well.

Swelling

An acute swelling or a high temperature may be associated with a dental infection and should be treated immediately. Any swelling in the body should be treated with suspicion and you should seek assistance straight away, but a swelling in the neck may be particularly dangerous because it can press against the airway as well as against the numerous blood vessels and nerves in this part of the body.

A dental infection can spread through the body very rapidly but, sometimes, the dentist can simply make a hole in the tooth so that the infective material actually drains away. This procedure will also relieve any pressure that has built up in the tooth as a result of the decomposition of the nerve and blood vessels and thereby relieve pain.

When infection enters the body, whether it is from bacterial or fungal organisms, or even by chemical means, the body's white blood cells are killed. Other chemicals, known as enzymes further break down the surrounding healthy tissue and the resulting creamy fluid is called pus. It is contained within a cavity to form an abscess. An abscess can burst spontaneously – you probably know what it is like to lance a boil. Incising is the clinical way of draining an abscess. The swelling caused by an abscess may not be painful and the most dependent part of it can be incised with a scalpel so that copious amounts of the foul-smelling pus are released. Minor surgery of this kind is not painful. The feeling of relief which comes when the abscess is incised is immense. To increase the body's resistance to the infective bacteria, the dentist may prescribe a course of antibiotics. Even if the infection responds very rapidly to this treatment, you should always complete the whole course of medication to prevent the bacteria from building up a resistance to the antibiotics. Only if there is an obvious allergic reaction to the antibiotic drug should you discontinue the course of treatment, and then you should return to your dentist to explain what has occurred.

An abscessed tooth is not always doomed to the surgery bucket, although it may be necessary to extract it when the swelling has subsided. It may be possible to treat the tooth and save it. Even if the infection stems from the gum rather than from the tooth itself, the tooth can still be retained. In this case, the area around the tooth would be thoroughly cleaned and scaled, and some periodontal surgery performed, but, again, the tooth may need to be root treated.

Treating yourself

We have already explained the treatment that is required to control the bleeding that may occur after a tooth has been extracted. If the bleeding continues you should only apply mechanical pressure to the socket and seek advice straight away. We must emphasize that there are no drugs used to control bleeding which you can safely administer yourself and you should not, under any circumstances, attempt to do so.

When you have painful teeth and gums, well-meaning people often suggest remedies to relieve your suffering. This condition requires expert attention, however, and we must condemn the application of almost all kinds of unprescribed pain-relieving substances. Some people might suggest that you should place an aspirin next to the aching tooth but this can be most injurious because aspirin contains salicylic acid which will burn the gum tissue. You will be left with a raw, reddened wound with folds of dead, white skin at its edges – it will look rather like the affects of sunburn. Aspirin is a very effective painkiller, however, when taken by mouth as directed but it is an irritant to the stomach and, ideally, should only be taken after meals. Paracetamol, on the other hand, is far less irritating to the stomach but, if taken in large doses, it is likely to cause liver damage, which does not become apparent until some four to six days after the dose has been taken. Ideally, as we have stressed all along, all drugs should only be taken on prescription from dentally or medically qualified practitioners.

Even the tooth tinctures that can be bought from chemists can irritate the gums if they are used to excess. But, as we have stressed throughout this book, painful teeth and gums require the correct dental treatment and you should never use any pain-controlling medication for more than a few hours, especially in the case of children.

Antibiotics treat infection and are not pain controllers. Even if the pain is caused by an infection, you must not be tempted to take a small dose of old penicillin tablets that you may have lying about the house. This is only likely to increase the bacteria's resistance to the antibiotic and, anyway, you should not have any drugs left over from a previous treatment in the first place. As a general rule to be strictly observed, you should always dispose of any unfinished medicines safely and sensibly, either by returning them to a chemist or to your doctor, if they are fairly new, or by flushing them down the lavatory. Even if you do have drugs in the house which were originally prescribed to treat dental pain, never use them for different episodes of dental problems.

You may find it helpful to apply clove oil to a painful tooth but, once again, you should not be content with this treatment for more than a day. You must make an appointment to see your dentist. In fact, clove oil mixed with white zinc oxide powder is actually used by dentists as a temporary dressing. (Could this be herbal dentistry?) The dressing hardens, keeping the clove oil in contact with the raw dentine, and does help to minimize the pain from the tooth. It is really very effective!

Dental pain requires dental treatment and, unfortunately, we cannot recommend drinking whisky or any other alcoholic beverage to control pain, even though it was used as an anaesthetic in the past. Alcohol will raise the blood pressure slightly and, if you have just had a tooth extracted, it may cause excessive bleeding from the socket.

We have already discussed the manufacture and fitting of dentures in a previous chapter but, if you do damage them, you should be able to find a dentist or a dental technician to carry out emergency repairs. It is even possible to buy products for denture repairs from some chemists and it is a good idea to include one of them in your emergency dental first aid kit which it is worth keeping in the house. Never use ordinary household adhesives to repair broken dentures for they often contain chemicals which, even after the glue has hardened, may irritate your mouth and damage your dentures.

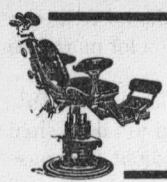

6 ORTHODONTICS – BELTS AND BRACES

Orthodontics is the name given to the branch of dentistry which deals with those conditions that result in a loss of chewing efficiency and/or the creation of an unacceptable appearance owing to the position of the teeth in the dental arches. Orthodontics is not an isolated speciality ·within dentistry but is an integral part of the whole subject. The need for orthodontic treatment is based on preventive, cosmetic, and functional considerations. The correction of a 'crowded dentition', for example, will facilitate adequate cleaning, particularly flossing.

According to a report published by the Welsh Office of the UK Department of Health and Social Security in 1973, more than 50 per cent of children have some kind of irregularity in their teeth. Of these, however, less than half need any kind of appliance (brace) to correct the problem – if it can be called a problem. We must stress that a deviation from what we might consider normal may not necessarily result in a loss of function nor the creation of an unacceptable appearance. Beauty is in the eye of the beholder!

The irregularities which can occur may interfere with the way the upper and lower teeth meet when the jaws are closed. A lack of contact in any region results therefore in a loss of chewing efficiency. The angulation of the teeth may lead to an unacceptable appearance, particularly in profile. Sometimes, these problems can be avoided by the well-timed extraction of some of the first teeth and, more commonly, the premolar teeth of the permanent dentition.

The pattern of meeting of the upper and lower teeth is referred to as the *occlusion* and, generally, the situation shown in Figure 3 is the normal arrangement. Deviations from this 'norm' are referred to as *malocclusions*. The way in which the various malocclusions are classified enables dentists to communicate with one another more easily but, just for the record, the norm is referred to as a Class I occlusion, although individual tooth malpositioning can occur even in this arrangement.

Class II describes the situation in which the upper teeth protrude in the incisor region *(see Figure 23)*. This condition can arise because of the undergrowth of the lower jaw, overgrowth of the upper jaw in the incisor region, or, in some cases, may also be caused by the habits of tongue thrusting, thumb sucking, or lip biting. Class III refers to the condition which exists when the lower incisor teeth are in front of the upper incisor teeth when the jaws are closed. This condition is commonly associated with overgrowth of the lower jaw bone. *(See Photo 20, lower models.)*

Even though the improvement in appearance which can be achieved by orthodontic treatment is not the only factor which dictates the need for treatment, orthodontics is probably the first introduction that many of us experience to what is, in essence, cosmetic dentistry. Indeed, it is often the look of a child's teeth and jaws that prompts parents to seek advice.

Despite some reports, and even the comments that we have made in this book on the effects that modern diet and other environmental factors have on the teeth, most dental derangements have been shown to be of genetic origin. These genetic variations can, therefore, result in disproportionate sizes of the teeth and jaws which lead to malocclusions and incorrect positioning of individual teeth. Though most dental irregularities of this kind are genetic in origin, we have also referred elsewhere to the possible effects of sucking habits on the dental arches. It is generally accepted that there is a connection between the development of the arches and the action of surrounding muscles which are those of the tongue and lips. The tongue is extremely strong and can exert considerable pressure on the front teeth – so much so that the teeth will eventually protrude. Placing the thumb in the mouth and sucking for long periods of time may further worsen an existing malocclusion. There is no direct evidence that tongue thrusting or thumb sucking actually cause a malocclusion but these habits almost certainly worsen a condition which already exists.

During a baby's first year, it may be that thumb sucking is due to dissatisfaction with breast feeding because the flow of milk to the baby is too fast but, more commonly, this is associated with bottle feeding. Decreasing the size of the hole in the teat of a bottle which is used to feed the baby will stimulate it to suck more. The instinct to suck in the newborn offspring of many species of mammals is particularly strong and we might even suggest that there is some sensory deprivation in babies who are not suckled correctly. We have already mentioned that preventive dentistry should begin at the antenatal stage, and this is as necessary for orthodontic reasons as it is for the prevention of gum disease and tooth decay. You should be careful not to scold a child for thumb sucking; the best approach is gently to move his or her hand away from the mouth and to try to occupy the child's attention with other toys. In older children, hypnosis has been used to attempt to break the thumb sucking habit. One report suggested that the children should be told that sucking the thumb alone was quite unfair, and that all the other fingers and the other thumb should receive equal attention. This would then become so tedious for the child that the habit is given up. If thumb sucking persists to an age at which the second dentition has erupted, the dentist can offer more practical help. Plates of different kinds can be fitted in the child's mouth but it is considered that this procedure is unacceptable for children under the age of five years.

An important factor in the development of malocclusions is the premature loss of some of the first teeth. Some parents assume that it is alright to lose some of the primary (milk) teeth because they feel these teeth are not important. This is quite wrong, however, and the first teeth are just as important as the permanent dentition. Premature loss of the first teeth can result in drifting and spacing of the other teeth which can lead to a malocclusion. Occasionally, when a tooth is lost, sadly through decay or accident, in a mouth where there is no other factor which could cause orthodontic problems, the dentist might suggest fitting a space maintainer. This is shown in Figure 22. It is only considered to be necessary if there is to be no extraction of permanent teeth for orthodontic reasons later.

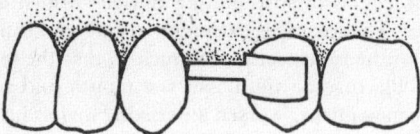

Fig. 22 A space maintainer – often short term. This simple space-maintaining device is fitted around the tooth and is maintaining space in the 4–5 region (upper left).

The restoration of decayed milk teeth is also important in space maintenance, and the teeth may even tilt or drift into a space created by the loss of just a part of a tooth. Thus, it is extremely important to conserve the primary dentition. Good oral hygiene, and the application of the preventive techniques mentioned in Chapter 2 is also important for orthodontic reasons.

Orthodontic treatment is only recommended where the end result will give a lasting improvement. Sadly, in some cases, a relapse occurs after much effort has already been made. If the improvement in the dentition which has been brought about by orthodontic treatment does last, then the procedures have been justified.

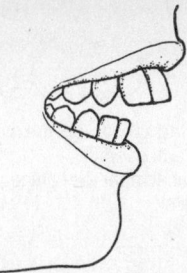

Fig. 23a   A malocclusion class II, division I – prominent front teeth. Note that the molars and canines in the upper jaw are in advance of the lower molars and canines.

An example of a common type of malocclusion is shown in Figure 23a and *see Photos 20, 1 & 2*. Occasionally, in this situation, the lower teeth actually bite into the palate at the back of the upper front teeth. The indentation formed by the tips of the lower teeth can ulcerate and become quite sore. The profile of a child with this problem is quite characteristic and school mates may tease the youngster.

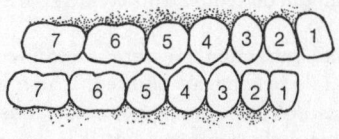

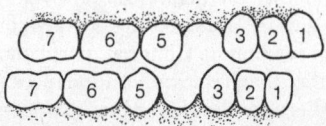

Fig. 23b   The class II malocclusion in profile. The first premolars are extracted (upper and lower 4s). The right side is shown here but the left side is similar and all four teeth are extracted.

The condition may be treated by removing the sound premolar teeth as shown in Figure 23b and a brace is then fitted to retract the upper canine teeth into the space created. The other front teeth are then aligned in the arch by the labial bow *(see Figures 23c & d)*. To balance the extractions, two lower teeth are often removed, too. Sometimes, molar

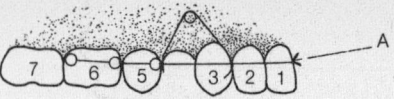

Fig. 23c An appliance is fitted to pull back the canine teeth, that is, the 3s are retracted using a canine retractor spring.
A   A labial bow is usually placed after the canines are back in the space occupied originally by the first premolars.

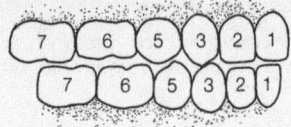

Fig. 23d An additional appliance then pulls back the four front teeth.

teeth, rather than premolars, are extracted, and the indications for extractions may also be based on the condition of the teeth. Usually, it is the first premolar teeth which are removed but if, for example, the second premolars were badly decayed or already had large restorations, then the dentist might be tempted to create space by extracting those teeth instead.

Where additional retraction pressure is required, appliances which fit around the child's head, may be used. These are called extra-oral traction appliances. Wearing an appliance of this kind may cause a sensitive child some embarrassment but it is hoped that the resulting improvement in appearance will be worth the upset.

The appliances shown in Figure 23c are referred to as removable appliances, and it is wise for a child to take them out if they take part in contact sports or in swimming. Children, particularly, may benefit from the use of fixed, rather than removable, appliances to move teeth into the required position. Because the child cannot remove the appliance, he or she will be obliged to keep it in place even at school. These appliances can be very comfortable but, because they cover most of the teeth, they are hardly attractive to look at. It is to be hoped that if the child understands that submitting to this for a few months will eventually result in an improvement of the dentition later, the brace will not need to be worn against the child's will. Of course, good oral hygiene must be maintained throughout the course of treatment.

Adults, even in middle age, may also have orthodontic treatment, although it is generally accepted that teeth move more quickly through young bone. To speed up the movement of teeth through the bone in adults, it is possible to carry out an operation, known as *corticotomy*, in which, under a general anaesthetic, the bone around each tooth is cut away. Braces are then fitted to the teeth, as usual, but the end result is achieved more quickly. Operations of this kind are normally carried out in hospital by a consultant orthodontist and/or an oral surgeon. It must be borne in mind that some orthodontic procedures may take as long as two years to be completed, and even moving only one tooth may involve three months' treatment followed by a period of retention.

It is possible that a malocclusion may be due to a gross abnormality of the bony development of the jaw. Many people may be worried by the appearance of their teeth and jaws, and your dentist may not wish to draw your attention to the problem for fear of upsetting you. If you are in any way concerned about such a condition, therefore, do ask your dentist about it because it is likely that it can be corrected. For example, even an extremely prominent lower jaw, such as the one of the young girl shown in the photo section, can be corrected by orthodontic treatment. Of course, the improvement in appearance, following an operation of this kind, will be considerable. In fact, the condition shown in the illustration is known as Hapsburg Jaw because it was a hereditary feature of that royal family. *See Photos 20, 3 & 4.*

Orthodontic treatment is a highy specialized and extremely important branch of dentistry and, with the improvement in oral hygiene so that we are better able to keep our teeth and gums healthy and free from decay and disease, it may become even more necessary and popular in the future. Remember that it may assist greatly in controlling plaque by reducing the crowding in the mouth and minimizing the areas of plaque stagnation. Bear in mind that orthodontic treatment should not be forced on children and that careful discussion with your child at home is extremely important. Indeed, it may well be worth making an initial visit to your dentist without your child to arm yourself with information that you can pass on to him or her.

The timing of orthodontic treatment is quite crucial, and a dentist will not want your child to wear an appliance for too long. Unless there is a fairly rapid initial improvement in the dentition, the child may well lose heart, and the removable type of appliance will spend more time on the child's desk at school than it does in the mouth. Fixed appliances do not have this disadvantage but, of course, they are usually only constructed where multiple, difficult tooth movements are to be carried out.

Your dentist may recommend that, even after treatment is complete, your child should continue to wear the appliance at night time only. Please make sure that you follow this advice to the letter. Relapse of orthodontic malocclusions, because the appliances were not retained long enough, are not uncommon. Orthodontic treatment using appliance therapy is normally begun in the child's eleventh or twelfth year but it is important to seek advice frequently before this age.

Clean the orthodontic appliance with a toothbrush and water. Instruct your child to fill a bowl of water and to clean the appliance over the bowl. If the child drops the appliance while cleaning it, then it will fall into the water and not break. In this way, valuable time and effort will not be wasted.

Tooth oddities

We have already mentioned in a previous chapter that some of the teeth may be partially absent. Sometimes, the spaces which result from this *partial anodontia* can create an unacceptable appearance or loss of function of the teeth. In some cases, this condition can be improved by the use of orthodontic appliances and partial dentures. In adults, sophisticated bridgework can be employed.

Some people have extra or *supplemental* teeth. These may cause crowding and may need to be extracted. Where there is extra dental tissue present in the mouth but it does not closely resemble the shape of the natural teeth, it is referred to as a *supernumary* tooth. Such teeth do not always erupt fully and may impede the eruption of the natural teeth. Photo 1 shows the appearance of a supernumary tooth in the midline – the so-called *mesiodens*. The supernumary was not causing pain but its presence was causing spacing between the two front incisors. Extraction of supernumary teeth is not a major operation but it does generally involve an overnight stay in hospital because a general anaesthetic is invariably needed.

When some of the first teeth are retained in the lower jaw and the permanent successors have already erupted, patients often become quite alarmed about this situation. There is no need to worry. The retained deciduous teeth are simply removed and, in most cases, there is no lasting damage to the dentition *(see Figure 24)*.

Fig. 24 Retained deciduous teeth. These can be extracted and the central incisors behind them will move forward in most cases into a favourable position. This usually occurs in six- to eight-year-olds.

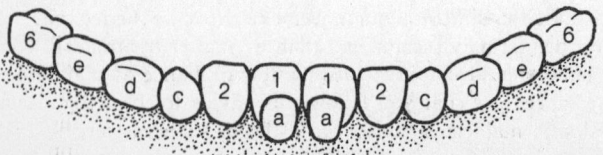

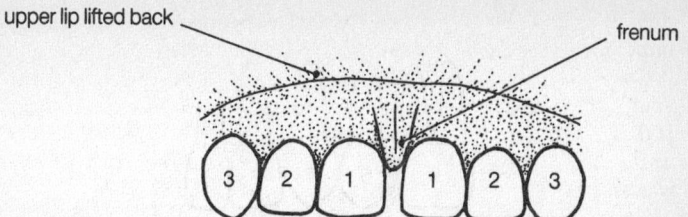

upper lip lifted back

frenum

3 2 1 1 2 3

Fig. 25 The labial frenum of fibrous tissue creating a midline space between the upper central incisors. The frenum can be removed surgically in a short operation, usually performed under a local anaesthetic only.

You will see that irregular tooth positions may be due to a variety of dental tissue abnormalities, and to undue pressure placed on the teeth by muscular activity, such as thumb sucking. A rare occurrence is the presence of an enlarged *fraenum*. This is the band of muscle and fibrous tissue which extends from the inner surface of the upper and lower lips to the gum between the front incisors *(see Figure 25)*. It may have an unacceptable appearance in itself but it also often maintains a space between two incisor teeth. This may be treated by reducing its size surgically under a local anaesthetic. If, however, there is spacing elsewhere in the dental arch, the space between the incisors may not close even if the frenum is reduced in size.

Where there is an obvious spacing present between teeth but there are no teeth missing, a radiographic examination may reveal cysts, tumours, or odontomes. Cysts are not uncommon in young people. Collections of cells, sometimes leftovers of development in the embryo, enlarge and absorb more fluid than the surrounding tissues giving rise to the formation of a cell-lined, fluid-filled cavity or cyst. To remove it, the patient may require a small operation under general anaesthesia.

Thankfully, tumours are quite rare but, obviously, they must not be overlooked and, once again, any dental abnormality should be investigated, even if only to eliminate this condition as a possibility.

Odontomes are bizarre collections of odd dental tissue. Sometimes, they are reminiscent of enamel, dentine, or cementum and sometimes mixtures of all these tissues. They are not dangerous but they may undergo cystic change to cause spacing of the teeth.

Gemination (twinning) may occur occasionally in the primary dentition, though not exclusively. In this condition, the crowns of the two teeth fuse together while they are forming and, although they occupy their usual position in the arch, they may appear to be slightly smaller than the total width they would have been, if they had appeared in the

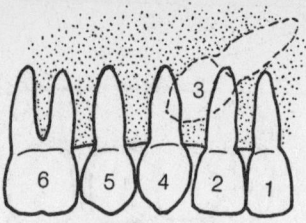

Fig. 26a An impacted canine tooth lying in the palate.

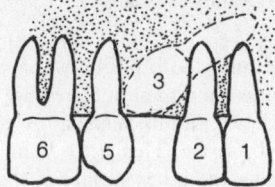

Fig. 26b The first premolar (4) is removed.

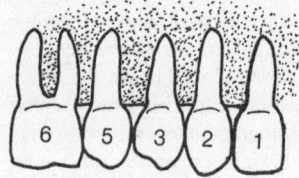

Fig. 26c A cap splint is fitted to the partially exposed canine (3) and is pulled into the space provided by the extraction of the 4. It may, however, erupt into the space of its own accord if it is more favourably placed.

usual way. They rarely require removal and, indeed, it is merely worth bearing in mind that the demarcation line between the two crowns may be a plaque trap.

Replanting teeth that have been lost in an accident is intended to maintain the correct spacing, and the orthodontic aspect of replacing such *subluxed* teeth should not be ignored. Another orthodontic procedure which is not uncommon is replanting teeth which have become buried in the jaw. One good example of this condition may occur with the upper canines, as is shown in Figures 26a, b & c. The canine tooth can remain totally unerupted and not cause any pain or discomfort. When it becomes necessary to pull this tooth into the arch because of the possibility of it causing problems later, the dental surgeon may extract the first premolar tooth, extract the canine, and replant it in the prepared socket of the premolar. Sometimes only the crown of the canine tooth is exposed, in which case a splint cap is fixed to the crown, and, using another tooth as an anchorage point, a system of wiring is used to pull the canine into its proper space.

You will have realized that orthodontics is not a line of treatment to be entered into lightly and it is worth remembering the following points:

1 Timing of the treatment is important.
2 All other aspects of dental care are just as important in orthodontic treatment as wearing an appliance.
3 The method used to feed your baby may affect the alignment of the teeth – sucking habits can worsen the condition.
4 The treatment may involve the extraction of healthy teeth to lessen crowding.
5 The condition may only be improved and not necessarily cured.
6 Take care not to impose your will on your children.

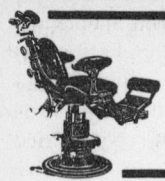

7 CONTROLLING PAIN

Anaesthesia in dentistry

The story of how methods have been used to control pain spans many centuries and even the Greek poet, Homer, refers in the *Odyssey* to certain medicaments which affect sensation and feeling. The ancient Egyptians used Cannabis Indica as an anaesthetic, while the Greeks were familiar with the use of extracts from poppy plants, and the Romans developed mixtures of herbs and other plants that would cause a deep sleep. In some cases, the purpose was that patients should be unable to feel pain during surgical operations. Indeed, throughout history, many people have contributed to our current knowledge of anaesthesia.

In 1681, a book was published which drew attention to the use of gases as a means of anaesthetizing patients. On 10 December, 1844, Gardner Q. Colton, a lecturer in surgery, spoke of the effects of nitrous oxide on the human body. One Samuel A. Cooley 'took the gas' and during the demonstration he bruised his legs and appeared to suffer no pain. This incident resulted in the dentist, Horace Wells, inviting Colton and another dentist, John Mankey Riggs, to perform a surgical extraction of a painful tooth. The patient was Wells himself. The tooth was extracted on 11 December, 1844 and Wells, fully recovered, reported that he felt no pain, nor was aware of the surgical procedure being carried out. On future occasions, Wells carried out this procedure in his own practice and the extraction of teeth under general anaesthetic was performed successfully on many patients. Wells was also familiar with the effects of the gas ether but he chose to use nitrous oxide. In 1845 Wells went to Boston, Massachusetts to bring nitrous oxide before the medical profession. He spoke to the class of John Collins Warren and tried to demonstrate the effects of nitrous oxide. In not giving his patient sufficient gas, or possibly attempting to extract the tooth too soon into the anaesthetic, the patient reeled in agony and the entire audience hissed and jeered at Wells. He returned to his home town of Hertford, Connecticut deeply discouraged and dejected. Meanwhile, Well's former partner in dental practice, William Morton had encountered much success using ether. In January 1847, Wells went to Paris and published a letter in the *Gallignani's Messenger* on 17 February, 1847 claiming priority for the use of the anaesthetic, nitrous oxide. Ether, however, was recognized to be a superior anaesthetic agent, though Wells tried desperately to prove nitrous oxide to be so. Wells moved to New York and experimented with other gases on himself. On one occasion, on 21 January, 1848, he became so deranged by the effects of some of these gases that he attacked a passer-by. He was arrested and imprisoned and, while there, on 24 January, 1848, inflicted a wound on himself which severed an artery in his thigh and he bled to death. On 25 January, 1848, these facts were unknown to the Paris Medical Society which that very day proclaimed Wells the discoverer of anaesthetic gases.

Anaesthesia had arrived and its advantages in surgery were recognized so that an eminent surgeon of the day, Mr Fergusson, reported in the second edition of his book, *Surgery*, 'It is, perhaps, not saying too much when this discovery is characterised as the greatest in most respects which has been made in the province of surgery.' Today, surgeons can painlessly transplant organs or carry out the most delicate operations without any discomfort to the patient.

Local anaesthesia only renders certain, localized parts of the body insensible to pain but it also has a long history. Most local anaesthetics used in dentistry are based on chemicals which are related to or associated with cocaine. Adrenaline is invariably added to the agent so that the blood vessels at the site of the injection constrict to keep the anaesthetic where it is meant to be. This also has the effect of reducing haemorrhage at the site of operation in case of surgery.

You will have gathered that there are two separate chemical ways of controlling pain during dental procedures:

1 General anaesthesia using the inhalation of gases, or the injection into the bloodstream of drugs which act on the brain and render the patient insensible to pain that way.

2 Local anaesthetics which act at the site of the surgery or which may be injected at some distance from the site to provide a regional anaesthetic or block.

It may be more straightforward to look at local anaesthesia first of all so that you will be able to appreciate why most of your mouth goes numb after you have had an injection for one filling in the lower jaw. *(See Figure 27.)* There is only one place where the main nerve trunk to the lower jaws and teeth is not surrounded by bone and this is at the corner of the

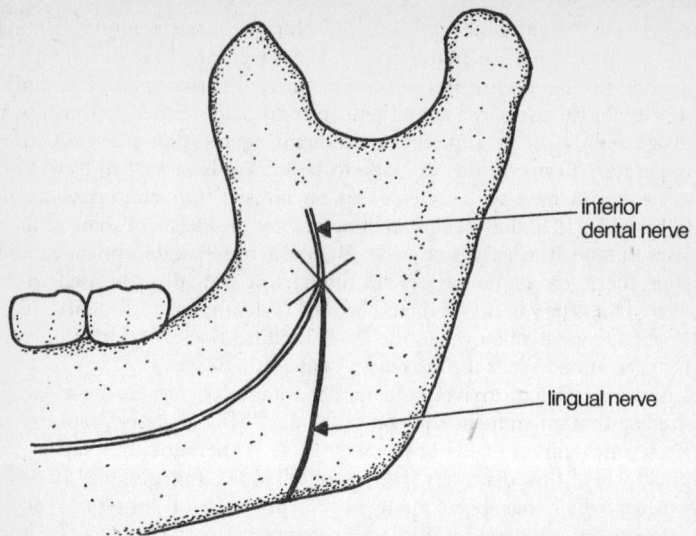

Fig. 27 The lower jaw, tongue side to show the point where the nerve enters the jaw bone. 'X' marks the spot where a local anaesthetic is inserted to make the tongue and lip numb. After this point the nerve to the teeth is within the jaw bone.

mouth where the nerve leaves its main trunk and enters the canal in the lower jaw bone. An injection of a local anaesthetic solution here will anaesthetize the lip, tongue, and gum, as well as the teeth, by a regional block. If a tooth is to be extracted from the lower jaw, the solution is also injected into the sulcus because there is another nerve supply here from a different source. Don't worry, then, if a good part of your mouth is affected after a couple of injections in the lower jaw – it is quite normal.

The upper teeth can also be anaesthetized by a regional block but it is more usual to use individual injections around each tooth that is to be treated or extracted. To make life even more comfortable, the dentist can now use local, topical anaesthetic creams so that you will hardly feel the prick of the needle. It still hurts you more than it does the dentist, however! It is important to remember that some anaesthetic solutions may interact with other drugs if the patient is taking any so you must give your dentist a full and complete medical history, including any medication that you are taking at the time.

As the law stands at the present, a general anaesthetic can be administered by a dentist, although the General Dental Council advises that all general anaesthetics should be given by a trained operator other than the operating dentist. If the dentist who is operating on you also accepts responsibility for administering the general anaesthetic, then you could be placing yourself at considerable risk possibly with fatal consequences. It is not a good idea to try to serve two masters and it is well-nigh impossible for the dental surgeon to function as the operator and the anaesthetist without jeopardizing one of the tasks in the process. If you or your child has to have a general anaesthetic for a dental operation, then make sure that there is a properly qualified person present for each part of the procedure. If you are in any way unsure, don't let the dentist go ahead, for you could be putting your or your child's life at risk by your consent. Do not allow yourself to be the patient of an operator-anaesthetist.

Ideally, dental operations involving the use of general anaesthetics should be carried out by experienced and properly qualified anaesthetists who have access to the equipment that might be needed in the case of an emergency. Only recently, deaths have been reported when a dentist acted as both the operator and the anaesthetist. The dentist was convicted of manslaughter, but this hardly compensates for the tragic death. Tragedy is never acceptable but it is made worse when it could have been avoided, particularly when an anaesthetic has been given to carry out a simple dental treatment.

It is permissible for a dentist to administer sedatives, such as Diazepam, provided a second, suitably trained person is present. A simple sedation may be defined as 'a technique in which the use of a drug or drugs produces a state of depression of the central nervous system, enabling treatment to be carried out, but, during which, verbal contact with the patient is maintained throughout the period of sedation. The drugs and techniques used should carry a margin of safety wide enough to render unintended loss of consciousness unlikely.' In other words, a sedative is a drug which calms the patient, so that he or she is willing and able to undergo surgery, but retains enough faculties to speak coherently and respond to commands. Inhaling certain anaesthetic gases, such as those administered during the early stages of childbirth, may also be considered as drugs of sedation, as are those which are injected into the arm veins of a patient for the same purpose.

Neither a sedative drug nor a general anaesthetic should ever be used on a patient if emergency equipment is not readily available. Recently, dentists have been advised that if they fail to comply with these directives, their conduct may be considered to be professionally infamous or disgraceful.

Warning

Prior to a general anaesthetic patients should have been starved of all food and drink for at least four hours and, in some cases, dentists may recommend six hours. No tight or restrictive clothing should be worn. All previous medical history should be made available to the dentist and his anaesthetist, particularly liver, heart, and chest trouble, and the taking of various drugs. After the anaesthetic, the patient should be accompanied by a responsible adult.

Alternative methods of pain control

Pain can be controlled by *hypnosis*. The word is derived from the Greek *hypnos* meaning sleep and the term was coined in the 1840s by a Scottish surgeon, James Braid. It was thought to have miraculous powers and it is likely that some aspects of witchcraft probably have a link with hypnosis. Hypnosis is a useful tool in dental surgery and it is unfortunate that its development was held up by its association with quackery.

The Austrian physician, Franz Anton Mesmer (1734–1815), found that some people attending his 'seances' appeared healed after he had waved magnets over them. It was then found that it was enough for people only to drink water over which he had passed a magnet. In Paris a Commission, which included the American diplomat, Benjamin Franklin (1706–90), and the French chemist, Antoine Laurent Lavoisier (1743–94), was set up to investigate his claims. In 1784, the Commission concluded that no 'magnetic fluid' existed and that the miraculous cures claimed to have been effected by Mesmer were due to imagination. They did not, however, deny that people had been cured.

Again, in about 1840, John Elliotson in London used hypnotism to practise surgery, including leg amputations, painlessly. Braid, however, separated the science of hypnosis from mesmerism and introduced the concept of monoideism, which is concerned with concentrating the focus of attention on one subject to the exclusion of all others. Even the Austrian psychoanalyst, Sigmund Freud (1856–1939), used hypnosis to treat some neurotic disorders. And, during the two World Wars, hypnosis was used in treating people suffering from the effects of shell shock and other neuroses. The earlier work resulted in the formulation of hypnosis as a state of hypersuggestibility, although there still remains no satisfactory theory of how hypnosis actually works.

The hypnotic state was a result of belief, misdirected attention, and expectation. In other words, it is an artificial state, resembling deep sleep, in which the person who has been hypnotized becomes involuntarily and unconsciously obedient to suggestions made by the hypnotist. Not everyone is susceptible to hypnosis, however, and anyone who is sceptical about its effects is less likely to be induced into a hypnotic state.

Hypnosis is not always successful in relieving pain, and its success does depend on the individual's pain threshold in the first place, but it can work very well so that even the most anxious person may allow surgery to be performed. It will help to eliminate stress and tension and allow the dentist to give an injection, for example, because the patient believes that it will not hurt. Indeed, cases have been reported in which teeth have actually been extracted with no other form of anaesthesia than hypnosis. Hypnosis can be particularly valuable in treating painlessly patients whose medical histories suggest that other, more conventional, anaesthetic techniques may not be advisable. Some patients worry about being placed in a hypnotic state in the belief that they will do or say something which they would not normally do and which may be embarrassing. It is unlikely, however, that anyone will do anything that is not normally in their nature. There is a London-based society, to which some dentists belong, that encourages the use of hypnosis in dentistry.

The suggestions of the hypnotist seem to be effective using a soft, monotonous voice describing scenes which allow a freedom of movement yet concentrate on one subject, such as a floating balloon. Really what is happening is that a focus of attention is being created to the exclusion of all other subjects. Under these circumstances, the pain threshold of the subject is modified, and many dentists have found that their patients show an increased pain threshold even under light hypnosis. Hypnotism is rarely used in major surgery but its use does enhance the effects of certain drugs. It can be used in childbirth and in the control of pain for untreatable terminal cancer patients. As well as for pain control, in dentistry, it is useful in suppressing the gagging reflexes and in helping people to adapt to new dentures.

As a science, hypnosis, like anaesthesia generally, is still in its infancy but the possibilities for its advancement are interesting and exciting. Unfortunately, however, because of its theatrical origins, the science of hypnosis has suffered a certain amount of ridicule. But, more will be learned about its function and effects as the pathways in the brain and the workings of the mind are uncovered. You must never try to practise hypnosis on one another but the use of suggestion should not be underrated. It may be particularly important in treating children. For example, if a child is told that the dentist is going to use a drill to prepare a tooth, he or she may expect to feel pain because his or her idea of a drill may be the one that is used to dig up the road. On the other hand, if when the dentist is preparing the tooth for a restoration, you need to explain the procedure, it is a good idea to associate what is happening with something pleasant. If, then, the dentist uses an instrument which creates a fine spray that is cold, like ice cream, try to persuade the child to think of the ice cream rather than about dentists' drills.

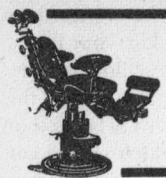

8 DRUGS, DISEASES, DANGERS, AND DENTISTRY

Some medical conditions, and the drugs that you may already be taking, as well as past medications or illnesses to which you have been subjected may have a significant bearing on any dental treatment that is planned for you. Some drugs, for example, interact with others that the dentist may use. Therefore, it is vitally important that you provide your dentist with a concise and accurate record of your current ailments or medications. Your dentist will treat this information in complete confidence and you should provide it freely.

You may be rather surprised by some of the questions that your dentist asks you because they may not seem relevant to dental treatment, but the diversity of problems which can affect the teeth and gums, as well as the treatment, is so wide that perhaps no-one knows the full implications of some conditions. So don't be shy; tell your dentist everything you know about your state of health. Some people are especially reticent about particular aspects of their health, such as sexually transmitted diseases, taking the contraceptive pill, taking antidepressant drugs, or even pregnancy. But it is important that your dentist should know about these subjects as we will discuss later in the chapter.

Heart conditions – rheumatic fever

This disease usually occurs in children between the ages of five and fifteen years and often follows a severe sore throat which has been caused by the bacteria streptococci. Rheumatic fever is referred to as an auto-immune disease which means that the body's reaction to infection is directed against normal, healthy body cells as well as against the affected ones. In the case of rheumatic fever, the joints and, sometimes, the heart valves may be damaged and, after the acute stage of the disease, the affected valves may remain damaged. The surfaces of the valves become roughened and the smooth flow of blood through the heart may be impeded, resulting in a heart murmur (abnormal heart sound).

Although not every case of rheumatic fever will result in damage to the heart valves, you must tell your dentist if you have ever suffered rheumatic fever because it is possible that, during dental procedures, such as the extraction of teeth, scaling, or extensive restorative treatment, the bacteria which normally live in the mouth may gain access to the bloodstream. Once they have entered into the circulatory system, these bacteria can set up infections in and around the heart valves. This may result in a serious, and possibly fatal, condition called endocarditis, which means an infection of the inner walls of the heart. Once this stage has been reached, using antibiotics may not be effective. Provided your dentist is aware of your condition, however, the problem can be avoided by the administration of antibiotics, such as penicillin or erythromycin, before dental treatment. In this way, the bacteria will be destroyed in the bloodstream before they can infect the heart valves and walls.

There are other conditions affecting the heart which your dentist should know about. These include congenital defects, such as a hole in the heart, Sydenham's chorea (St Vitus's Dance), and, of course, any history of heart operations, particularly the placement of artificial valves or pacemakers. Conversely, patients who are about to undergo heart surgery should certainly have a thorough dental examination and should be fully instructed in oral hygiene as part of their treatment.

Blood

An adult weighing about 70 kilograms (11 stones) has about 5 litres (8 pints) of blood coursing through the veins and arteries. Blood carries nutrients to various parts of the body and, in particular, conveys oxygen from the lungs to those tissues, such as muscles and the brain, which need the oxygen to be able to function. The oxygen is carried by the red blood cells in the blood, combining with the haemoglobin to form oxy-haemoglobin. It is the arterial blood which carries the oxygen while the blood flowing through the veins carries blood back to the heart once it has given up its oxygen. Obviously, any interference with the oxygen-carrying capacity of the blood is important. In dentistry, care must be taken when antibiotics are administered because these drugs may reduce the amount of oxygen which is available to the body and, therefore, your dentist must be aware if you suffer from any conditions, such as anaemia, which result in a low level of haemoglobin. Indeed, if your dentist feels that you need to be treated under a general anaesthetic, he or she may insist that you have a blood test first to make sure that your haemoglobin level and red blood cell count are normal.

Patients from Africa, the West Indies, Asia, or from Mediterranean areas may suffer from sickle cell anaemia and they should always be willing to have a specific blood test to check for this condition. Any reduction in oxygen in this condition may cause the blood cells to change from the normal saucer shape to a sickle shape, seriously reducing their capacity to carry oxygen and ultimately causing the cells to rupture. When this takes place, the bone marrow is unable to replace the red cells quickly enough and the condition may result in rapid death. Consequently, any procedures which may lower the potential oxygen which is available should only be carried out after testing for sickle cell anaemia. Of course, it is reassuring anyway, to know that your dentist has a record of whether you are sickle cell positive or negative, especially if you have to undergo dental or surgical procedures in the future. Patients should also be tested before any sedative techniques are used.

In 1925, Cooley and Lee described a severe type of anaemia called thalassaemia. Many of the patients were of Mediterranean origin and the disease is characterized by a decrease in the rate of production of the oxygen-carrying pigment, haemoglobin. The type of haemoglobin varies from the normal. The patients exhibit bone changes (bossing – enlargement of some skull bones) which may result in a malocclusion. The patients also seem to have an increased predisposition to infection. The disease leads to problems when the availability of oxygen is diminished, as may be the case under general anaesthesia.

You will have gathered that your dentist should know if you are suffering from any kind of anaemia. The elderly, the pregnant woman, or the nursing mother may be anaemic.

Haemophilia is an inherited blood disorder in which its ability to clot is impaired so that even minor wounds bleed uncontrollably. It affects about six people in every 100,000. Haemophilia arises because the body is unable to produce a substance called blood factor 8 which is referred to as antihaemophiliac globulin or AHG. Other factors responsible for blood clotting may also be deficient as is the case in patients suffering from a condition known as Christmas Disease. Patients suffering from these diseases can be treated, usually in hospital, by the administration of particular blood factors. Obviously, extracting teeth from haemophiliacs is likely to be hazardous and best avoided, so that dental disorders should be prevented, if at all possible, and it is vital that these patients should be thoroughly instructed in good oral hygiene techniques.

A blood test may also reveal deficiencies in the white blood cells which are largely responsible for the control of infection in the body. It is also possible that the body may be producing many abnormal, immature white blood cells, which is one of the characteristics of leukaemia, which disease may show other symptoms in the mouth. Severe ulceration and bleeding of the gums are most likely to be the result of poor oral hygiene but, if these problems persist in a clean mouth, they should be investigated promptly.

Lungs

Sometimes, lung infections can give rise to halitosis (bad breath) and your dentist might well bear this in mind if you complain that you are suffering from this embarrassing condition because, in the absence of dental disease, it is a likely cause of the problem. We have already mentioned the importance of anaemia, when anaesthetics are administered and, similarly, the efficiency of the lungs is of paramount importance in the absorption of oxygen. Therefore, you should always tell your dentist if you have recently had a bad cough, cold, influenza, or any other chest infection, such as tuberculosis, pleurisy, or pneumonia. Obviously, if you were suffering from one of these diseases, you would be unlikely to have a general anaesthetic for dental work but, if your dentist is aware of the situation, it might well influence any decision that the dentist or anaesthetist may come to for future treatment.

Brain

Mental handicap presents a particular problem in dental treatment because today's dentistry does depend largely on communication between dentist and patient. Therefore, any mentally handicapped person must be made aware, if at all possible, of the importance of good preventive measures. This aspect of prevention is dependent mainly on strengthening the enamel, that is, by fluoridation administered both systemically (in water or tablet form) and topically by the application of gels, and on the control of the sugar, particularly sucrose, in the diet of the handicapped person. Often mentally handicapped children and adults are treated under general anaesthetic and, although it is not uncommon for general dental practitioners to treat such patients, many are dealt with in a hospital environment.

Brain damage after an accident may result in mental as well as physical handicap. In the case of a physically handicapped person, the electric toothbrush may well prove to be very useful and people with orthopaedic injuries should be reminded that, with limited hand movements, the maintenance of good oral hygiene may require additional time and effort.

The brain may be damaged when a blood clot blocks a blood vessel supplying part of the brain. This is commonly referred to as a stroke. The side of the face may be partially paralyzed as well as the hand and leg on one side of the body. Obviously, food debris is likely to accumulate in the sulcus of the mouth on that side due to lack of tongue and lip movement. When the patient has recovered sufficiently, this should be pointed out so that additional effort to clean the area can be made.

Depression, as a result of a stressful situation such as severe domestic problems, may result in bruxism (grinding of the teeth) and a lack of personal hygiene which may cause an increase in tooth decay and gum disease. It is possible that social workers can help here by bringing the problem to the attention of such a person if the situation permits.

In the case of the condition known as hydrocephalus, where the fluid surrounding the brain does not drain away normally, a special device or shunt may be fitted to aid the drainage. As with artificial heart valves, these appliances may encourage the stagnation of bacteria and the patient may need to be treated with antibiotics before any dental work is carried out. Again, all such children must be taught good oral hygiene and the sugar intake should be controlled.

In epilepsy part of the brain is damaged, although this does not infer a reduced mental capacity. Epileptics are often treated using a drug called phenytoin sodium, which has the unfortunate side effect of causing the fibrous tissue parts of the gums to enlarge, possibly requiring corrective surgery. On the other hand, periodontal specialists generally feel that, if plaque is properly controlled, epileptics are less likely to require this form of treatment.

Nervous system

There are some disorders of the nervous system which diminish a person's response to pain. For example, a child with chronically carious teeth but with no apparent pain may be a sufferer, although this condition is rare. A much more common and localized condition is Bell's Palsy, first described by Sir Charles Bell (1774–1842) whose book, *Nervous Systems of the Human Body*, published in 1830, was well received by his contemporaries. Bell's Palsy usually affects one of the facial nerves which supply the muscles of facial expression in one side of the face. This condition can arise quite suddenly and may be distressing. Sometimes, the palsy is caused by pressure on the nerve from injury, tumour, or infection but, more commonly, it arises spontaneously as in true Bell's Palsy.

If you are affected by the condition, you should visit your medical practitioner straight away so that anti-inflammatory drugs, known as steroids, may be prescribed for you. It seems that the quicker the treatment is begun, the shorter the time that the nerve is affected and a return to normal is possible. Patient's suffering from Bell's Palsy may drool saliva from the corner of the mouth and the lip may droop on one side, but the dentist should be able to help here if the patient is a denture wearer by increasing the bulk of the denture to give more support to the cheek. Even where the natural dentition is present, the dentist can fit an appliance to the cheek side of the teeth on the affected side which carries a roll of plastic to support the cheek. The patients gain great comfort from the improvement to their appearance, so a trip to the dentist may be invaluable.

Kidneys

The kidneys assist in the excretion from the body of certain toxic waste products. Persistently taking drugs may damage the kidneys and, indeed, paracetamol, aspirin, and caffeine have all been implicated if they are taken over a prolonged period. Older people, in particular, may suffer from impaired kidney function so that the dosages of any drugs may need to be modified to take this into account. Patients on dialysis machines may be fitted with arterio-venous shunts to assist the fixing of tubes to the veins and arteries. These shunts may be left attached after dialysis and, as in the case of the shunts used in the treatment of hydrocephalus, they may become a hiding place for bacteria.

A dentist may provide antibiotic cover for these patients as a precaution in case the dental procedure itself results in the introduction of bacteria into the bloodstream. In these circumstances this would almost certainly be carried out in conjunction with advice from the patient's physician.

Liver

The liver destroys toxins and helps to remove waste products from the body. One particular transmissable disease, hepatitis, is especially hazardous to your dentist, staff, and other patients. The virus which causes the disease may be found in saliva as well as blood and many patients suffering from hepatitis are treated in special centres, Drug addicts may contract hepatitis from using dirty needles, and there is probably a case for compulsory registration of all tattoo artists and ear-piercing clinics to ensure that proper sterilization of equipment is carried out. It has been reported that the virus associated with the Acquired Immune Deficiency Syndrome is occasionally present in saliva. There is obviously a need, therefore, for some directive to patients, medical and dental practitioners where the disease is reported to be prevalent, when dental treatment becomes necessary, even a simple dental examination.

Alcohol, too, affects the liver resulting in a condition known as cirrhosis, and past and present alcoholics may suffer from liver damage. If you know that you have been affected in this way, you must tell your dentist because any future drug therapy or treatment may need to be modified.

Diabetes

Diabetics are no more prone to tooth decay and gum disease than any other individuals but their healing capacity after injury or disease may be affected. Oral hygiene instruction and dietary control go hand in hand so there is every reason for a diabetic to be fully familiar with the methods of preventive dentistry.

Pregnancy

Most doctors of medicine and dentists agree that general anaesthetics, medications of any sort, and surgery or radiological procedures should be avoided for pregnant women patients. Local anaesthetics can be used, however, and some dentists recommend the use of a type which does not contain any adrenaline. It is during the first and final stages of pregnancy that medication in particular should be avoided and it is generally agreed that the middle three-month period is a safer time to provide treatment if it is essential. Antibiotics and tranquillizers should be rigorously avoided.

As almost every woman knows, pregnancy itself affects the hormone balance of her body. Such hormonal changes may possibly lead to an increased tendency towards gum disease although, if plaque build-up is properly controlled, this should not be a serious problem. Sometimes, however, the gum in a localized area may become extremely overgrown, resulting in a 'pregnancy epulis'. An epulis refers to any swelling on the gum and such may require removal surgically. The pregnancy epulis may disappear spontaneously after the birth of the child. If it is removed surgically it is easily carried out under local anaesthesia.

Anaemia, stress, and possibly morning sickness during pregnancy are factors to which more attention should be paid. Morning sickness may result in the regurgitation into the mouth of food from the stomach. This can have a damaging affect on the teeth because the regurgitated stomach contents are very acidic. Therefore, the mouth should be cleaned and rinsed after any episode of vomiting.

Menopause

Menstruation in women generally ceases between the ages of 45 and 55 years and may result in some oral symptoms, such as a dry mouth, or ulceration of the gums and other mucous membranes that line the mouth cavity. Abnormal taste patterns may also develop. These conditions may lead to extreme discomfort and difficulty in wearing dentures. Of course, a dry mouth also indicates a reduced flow of saliva so that acidity in the mouth may not be neutralized and decay of the tooth enamel may begin. Your dentist might suggest that hormone therapy prescribed by your medical practitioner could be useful. Local treatment of the condition may only be palliative. Owing to psychological disturbance at this time, a woman may habitually and painfully grind her teeth in her sleep – this is nocturnal bruxism. A bite guard may prove useful here.

Ulcers

An ulcer is a break in the skin or other lining material of the body. Such a lesion in the stomach, for example, is referred to as a gastric ulcer and may result from excess acidity eroding the stomach lining or, more recently, it has been suggested that it is caused by a virus. In the mouth, small ulcers, which can be extremely painful in the early stages, often develop at times of stress, such as during menstruation, and young girls beginning menstruation frequently experience ulceration of the tongue, cheeks, and gums. Any young person, taking school examinations or starting a new job, may suffer from ulcers, and adults can be affected, too. These aphthous ulcers, as they are called, have a yellowish surface with a raised and inflamed edge.They are rarely more than 0.5 centimetre long and are quite harmless, lasting for about eight days. An ulcer which persists for more than about a week, however, should be examined by your dentist or doctor. If you are particularly prone to ulceration of the mouth, you may get some relief from the application of an antiseptic gel to its surface; or your doctor or dentist may prescribe an anti-inflammatory drug to ease the condition. In any case, you certainly won't drown your fish and chips in vinegar!

Cold sores are caused by the herpes virus which may also affect other parts of the body. The virus lies dormant within the cells of the body, and it is only when you are subjected to further stress or illness that the familiar cold sore on the lips appears. When you first feel the typical burning sensation, it is well worth paying a visit to your doctor or dentist because you may be able to avoid the full effects of a cold sore by applying a medication to your lips when it first begins. Children sometimes suffer from a primary herpes infection which may affect the whole of the lining of the mouth. The gums often become red and painful, and many ulcers break out in the mouth. The child should rest in bed, and doctors and dentists usually recommend a diet of soft, nutritious foods which are low in sucrose – this is not an occasion for lack of plaque control! This condition should only last two or three days at most, and mouthwashes are often prescribed to prevent bacteria from infecting the ulcerated surfaces of the mouth.

A word of warning seems in order here. If you find that you have any kind of swelling or lumps and bumps in your mouth, or anywhere else for that matter, don't just sit back and hope they will go away. Seek medical or dental advice straight away. Not every little lump which appears spontaneously is likely to be dangerous but it is better to be safe than sorry; prompt treatment can even save lives in some cases.

Speech defects

Children who lisp or have some other speech impediment may also benefit from good dental care. Speech therapists are fully aware that certain sounds cannot be made properly without the use of the teeth, and dental defects, such as an open bite, will cause a speech difficulty. Underdevelopment of the lower jaw, for example, may result in the child having a lisp.

Denture wearers, also, may only be too aware of the effects of restricted tongue space on their speech patterns, and anyone who plays a musical wind instrument may find it difficult to cope with dentures. Fortunately, there are dentists who specialize in dental care for musicians but any budding wind instrumentalist or singer would do well to know about the way in which dental disease can play havoc with the voice or with the embouchure (the correct application of the lips and tongue in playing).

The voice is also dependent upon the bones around the face because spaces within them, called sinuses, affect its resonance. Anyone who has suffered with a heavy head cold knows what it is like to speak with that 'blocked-up' feeling. The sinuses in the upper jaw bones are very large. These sinuses can fill with mucus and inflammatory fluids causing the pressure within the sinus to be raised slightly. The lining of the sinus is close to the surface of the upper molars so that, when this happens, any movements of the head may cause pain in the teeth. This condition is known as sinusitis. The sinus in the upper jaw is also referred to as the antrum and it increases in size as the jaws develop. When an upper molar tooth is extracted, the dentist must be very careful not to push its roots into the antrum although, even if this does occur, it can still be retrieved but it requires a special surgical approach.

Ageing

Father time is no respecter of dental tissues and older people may be

108

presented with particular dental problems. We have already mentioned that kidney function is impaired in the elderly and that prescribing drugs is only undertaken with caution.

Over the years, tooth enamel is worn down by attrition and the individual's diet is perhaps the most important factor in the wear process. This wearing away of the enamel can occur at the contact points because, in time, the teeth may move slightly and rub against one another. Indeed, it has been reported that a one centimetre loss in the length of the dental arch can occur by the age of forty years.

Dentine continues to be produced throughout life and this has the effect of narrowing the pulp canals of the teeth. This makes root canal therapy (endodontic treatment) particularly difficult in the elderly. The extra dentine is called secondary dentine and is common in the aged. The tubules in the dentine may become sealed at one end and appear opaque to transmitted light. This has the effect of making the teeth look darker.

The pulp of the tooth changes with age. Sometimes, a pulp stone, which is a calcified nodule in the pulp canal or chamber, is seen. These pose problems for endodontic procedures.

The cementum, which covers the roots of the teeth, may increase with age but gum disease and the stresses of mastication may hinder its production. Sometimes, cementum becomes so abundant that extraction of a tooth becomes hazardous and a surgical approach is therefore necessary. It is wise to have radiographic pictures taken before a tooth is extracted if people are beyond middle age.

Becoming 'long in the tooth' is not entirely avoidable but it is likely that good oral hygiene throughout life, carefully planned dental treatment, and adequate nutrition may well result in a slowing down of the ageing effects in the gum and periodontal fibres, particularly by reducing stress in the biting surfaces of the teeth. Examination of teeth gives some indication of age and forensic scientists often use dental evidence to ascertain the ages of unidentified corpses. Wear patterns, pulp chamber thickness, and the colour changes in the dental tissues are used in the process of identification.

Artificial joints

Artificial joints, such as hip replacements, may provide a site for bacteria to lodge. As bacteria may enter the blood stream in dental surgery it is necessary, therefore, in some cases, to provide antibiotic cover for such patients before treatment. Though arthritis and rheumatism are not necessarily associated with old age, it is worth remembering that oral hygiene is affected by lack of manual dexterity.

Hereditary and birth defects affecting teeth and jaws

During the development of the face in the embryo, defects may occur which result in the formation of clefts, and lead to conditions such as a cleft palate or a hare lip. There is no evidence, however, that children suffering from these problems have weaker teeth or gums than others. Because they are diagnosed immediately nowadays, treatment to repair defects of this kind will often be started soon after birth. The growth of the teeth and jaws must be constantly supervised so that the right sort of corrective surgery and orthodontic treatment can be provided at the most suitable time. In the late 1970s, a breakthrough was made in detecting accurately changes which occur in body structure. Professor Peter Burke of Sheffield and Dr Leonard Beard of Cambridge University pioneered a system which can map, quite clearly, curves of the human body to an accuracy of 0.5 millimetre. In this way, a series of pictures can show how the soft tissue of the face can alter over a period of time, as well as indicating the effects of any corrective procedures.

Medicines

We have mentioned medicines elsewhere in the text but it is as well to be reminded that medicines which have been highly sweetened with sucrose are to be avoided if possible. Medication in pregnancy, in the elderly, and in those suffering from kidney and liver disease needs careful consideration. Some drugs affect the teeth of an unborn child. The antibiotic drug, tetracycline, crosses the placenta and causes yellow staining of teeth and bone. The approximate age at which the drug was administered can be determined from the position of the yellow band on the teeth which were forming at the time. Tetracycline is best avoided during pregnancy for this reason alone. Both first and second teeth may show staining for no apparent reason but, if there is a defect which stretches across several teeth, it is usually related to some interference in the growth and calcification process of the teeth. Measles, chicken pox, or any other bacterial or viral infection can upset the development of the teeth. Fortunately, however, any teeth that have been affected in this way can be crowned or coated with a veneer of tooth-coloured, plastic-like material, such as those used in the acid-etching technique mentioned in Chapter 3.

Another drug of interest, particularly to the mother-to-be, is metronidazole, which is often prescribed for gum infections and in post-operative care. This drug is partially secreted in breast milk and will therefore be passed on to the newborn child who clearly does not need it.

You should keep a record of all long-term medication and particularly steroids, anticoagulants, and drugs used in some mental disorders, such as mono-amine oxidase inhibitors and tricyclic antidepressant drugs. If you are taking any of these drugs, your medical practitioner will issue you with a blue card, such as the one illustrated in Figure 28. You must show these cards to your dentist and you should inform him or her if you have used the drugs within the previous two years.

If you do require dental treatment, it is possible that the dosage of steroids may need to be increased while antidepressant drugs may interact with some of the adrenaline-like compounds in local and general anaesthetics. Antidepressants are surprisingly widely used. Indeed, a recent report stated that one in five women and one in ten men take some kind of tranquillizer, and a total of twenty-five million prescriptions for drugs, such as diazepam, librium, and mogadon, are issued every year.

I am a patient on –

STEROID

TREATMENT

which must not be

stopped abruptly

and in the case of intercurrent illness

may have to be increased

INSTRUCTIONS

1 DO NOT STOP taking the steroid drug except on medical advice. Always have a supply in reserve.

2 In case of feverish illness, accident, operation (emergency or otherwise), diarrhoea or vomiting the steroid treatment MUST be continued. Your doctor may wish you to have a LARGER DOSE or an INJECTION at such times.

3 If the tablets cause indigestion consult your doctor AT ONCE.

4 Always carry this card while receiving steroid treatment and show it to any doctor, dentist, nurse or midwife whom you may consult.

5 After your treatment has finished you must still tell any new doctor, dentist, nurse or midwife that you have had steroid treatment.

Fig. 28 A Steroid Warning Card. (Crown Copyright. Reproduced with the kind permission of the Controller of Her Majesty's Stationery Office.)

The contraceptive pill

The contraceptive pill inhibits ovulation and, therefore, it disrupts the hormonal balance of the body. A girl may experience an increase in breast size, for instance, while taking the pill. The gums may be more susceptible to irritation by plaque in such a person, just as they are in pregnancy. It has been reported that the prescribing of some antibiotics may affect the efficacy of the contraceptive pill – this book is concerned with 'prevention' so don't forget to tell your dentist if you are taking the pill! It has also been reported that taking the pill over a long period of time may affect the heart and, more recently, a risk of cancer has been associated with some contraceptive pills. Fortunately, this has been brought to the public's attention.

Malignancy

As we have already explained, radiotherapy does have a bearing on the capacity of tissues, such as bone, to heal. Consequently, if you have had radiotherapy treatment to the head or neck, it is very important to avoid the need for dental surgery. Radiotherapy also affects the salivary glands. You may, therefore, experience a dry mouth as the production and flow of saliva, which tends to neutralize mouth acids, is reduced by the radiotherapy. There is, therefore, a greater risk of tooth decay. Mouthwashes may be helpful in reducing this risk and, because they often contain glycerine and thymol, your mouth will feel much more comfortable, too.

On the other hand, radiotherapy can actually be used to treat malignant disease of the jaws, tongue, lips, cheeks, and gums. At this point, it seems appropriate to mention again the risks associated with drinking alcohol and smoking. Smoking, drinking alcohol, or even eating highly spiced foods may not necessarily cause cancer of the soft tissues of the mouth, but a malignant change can certainly be exacerbated further by these habits. There is certainly, for example, a higher incidence of lip cancer among pipe smokers and there also seems to be a combined effect to increase the risk of cancer to those who smoke and also drink alcohol to excess.

If you smoke a pipe, it may be a good idea to inspect your mouth using a mouth mirror from time to time. You may notice that the roof of your mouth becomes very white and that small red dots appear. This is caused by the tiny glands in the roof of the mouth becoming blocked by the overproduction of the material keratin. The condition is called smoker's keratosis. It is not in itself a malignant condition and very few cases become so. You should, however, immediately cut down on your smoking and seek medical or dental advice. It is a sign that your smoking habit is affecting the health of your mouth. Even malignant conditions can be treated successfully if they are caught in time, so don't hesitate.

112

Fainting

Generally speaking, most people regard all dental treatment as an ordeal, although it should be no more so than any other kind of surgery. Perhaps it is the thought of the invasion of the mouth with needles and other metal paraphernalia which causes so much anxiety. In any case, fainting in the dental surgery cannot be considered to be a rare occurrence. It is caused by a temporary fall in blood pressure, possibly brought on by fear. Provided a faint is not prolonged, the patient should come to little or no harm but, if you know that you are prone to fainting at the sight of blood or a needle, then you should make sure that you are accompanied when you go for dental treatment. Certainly, if you have to have transport to reach the surgery and you are a car driver, don't be tempted to drive yourself home afterwards. Either arrange for a taxi to collect you or ask someone to accompany you on public transport. Your judgement may be impaired after a faint, so don't take any chances.

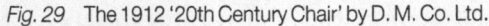

Fig. 29 The 1912 '20th Century Chair' by D. M. Co. Ltd.

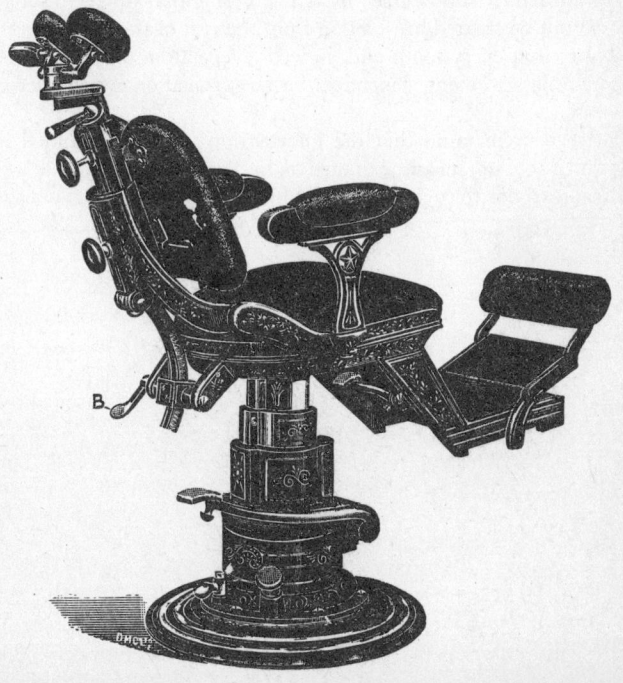

Changing your dentist

Multiple surgery practices may engage the services of different dentists. We feel that it is important to record the name of the dentists that have treated you and check that the new dentist is aware of any past medication and your medical condition. This particular aspect of dental care is quite worrying to patients and many do not like to see a succession of locums, associates, and assistants. This is quite understandable but often unavoidable. The advantages are that you may get the benefit of various opinions but the overriding disadvantage is a possible lack of continuity of care and that your new dentist may not initially be aware of your particular needs. With thorough questioning by the dentist and a patient freely giving personal information, the problem diminishes.

In conclusion

To practise dentistry, a person must be highly trained as well as having a wide knowledge of health care in general. Therefore, you can do a lot to help your dentist and yourself by remembering that the teeth should not and cannot be treated in isolation from the rest of the body. It is worth repeating that every tooth and, indeed, every atom of the body is, to a greater or lesser extent, dependent for its survival on every other part of the body.

Please bear in mind that the information we have included in this chapter is by no means exhaustive because it would need a whole medical textbook to cover the subject fully.

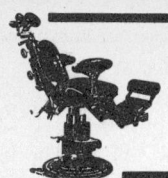

9 THE SHAPE OF TEETH TO COME

Throughout this book, we have emphasized that prevention is better than cure in dentistry. And, for everyone concerned with health care, there should be just one hope in their minds: that prevention of disease will become a reality. We are not there yet; a lot of work remains to be done and there is much to teach the young and old. As the tide is already turning and quite quickly now in favour of the preventive approach, more dental practices will be engaging the services of dental hygienists and personnel associated with dental health education. Let us hope that augmenting the speed with which the 'dental good news' is spread is associated with an increase in employment of people trained to pass on this information. Restorative dentistry for the treatment of tooth decay is likely to remain with us for many years to come, however, and will probably always be required for repairing traumatized teeth. Remember that, as we have explained, restorative dentistry is likely to be more effective and long lasting if plaque is controlled. Periodontal tissues in particular depend on the body as a whole to remain healthy. Therefore, the concept of whole body health needs further emphasis.

As we keep our teeth for longer and longer, the jaws may tend to become more crowded so that some types of orthodontic treatment will become more common. On the other hand, as decay is reduced and fewer and fewer teeth are lost prematurely, the mouths of more young people will have the chance to develop with a satisfactory occlusion so that less orthodontic work will be required to rectify other types of malocclusions. For older people, there is hope, too. As surgery techniques improve and quicker and quicker ways of treating adults with orthodontic needs are found, people who may now feel that it is too late to bother about their teeth may have the chance to enhance the appearance of their dentition.

Many factors, such as vaccine research, sugar substitutes, and, of course, the often-mentioned oral hygiene, are vital to maintain sound teeth and gums but perhaps the most important of all is a real desire, among everyone, to keep their own natural teeth all their lives. The overall importance of having good teeth and gums should be the point that is emphasized, perhaps by well-designed advertising in the media. We hope that, in future, government information services will be persuaded to promote dental health measures more frequently and more forcefully. In the UK, for example, some doctors have set up discussion groups with the help of the Royal College of General Medical Practitioners to which patients come and ask questions that might not be asked during a normal surgery consultation. We certainly believe that it would benefit dentists and patients alike if a similar scheme were to be adopted by the dental profession on an informal basis and at local level, so that many of the problems which worry patients could be cleared up.

There are still hurdles to be overcome, however. Reluctantly, we have to confess that dentists themselves are sometimes a little slow to accept change. In 1973, for example, the designer Richard Satherley won the Melchett award for designing the steel mobile dentistry unit which is illustrated in Photo 6 and reproduced with his permission. It consisted of a central column which carried air, water, and electrical services and which supported three rotary storage units made of plastic-coated steel. This particular design of equipment, which would help to reduce anxiety by its appearance and give the dentist a more comfortable environment in which to work, would be welcomed. It is a pity that cost is such an important factor in the choice of dental equipment. In the United Kingdom, for example, it may be the fee structure operating in the National Health Service which discourages some dentists from choosing such equipment. Many practices are extremely well equipped but, in some quarters, there is a reluctance to update.

Perhaps when the dental profession moves away from the 'item for a fee' approach, it will be encouraged by the fee structure itself not to choose equipment primarily on the basis of cost. It is important that the dental surgery should be designed to create an atmosphere which is pleasant and relaxing. In the photograph the way in which the instruments are thoughtfully and discretely hidden on the unit should reassure an apprehensive person. If for no other reason, there should be a change in the way that dentists are remunerated for their work so that they can operate in attractive surroundings with well-designed equipment to the benefit of dentist and patient alike. The authors hope that Richard Satherley's and other effective designs will become more widespread in British dental surgeries. We have also included an illustration from the 1912 catalogue of the Dental Manufacturing Company which shows the earlier 'twentieth century chair'. No doubt you will agree that it is a most interesting item of furniture and it probably did its job extremely well at the time but methods of dental care and treatment have changed and equipment should continue to develop, too. *(See Figure 29 & Photo 6.)*

116

There are many disciplines involved in dentistry and many discoveries yet to be made. We hope this book has revealed something of the science and that there is more to it than looking into mouths all day, as well as showing that the dental surgery should hold few terrors for anyone, especially if they care about the welfare of their teeth and gums.

Considering future trends in dentistry, we obviously hope that attitudes will change. A start has already been made and we have mentioned earlier the concept of whole body health which should include teeth and gums. On a more practical level, changes in attitude are only likely to be brought about through media publicity on the same scale as the anti-smoking campaign waged in the press and on radio and television. Bearing in mind the importance of diet on the health of the dentition, it would be a good idea if all foodstuffs were clearly marked to indicate the levels of sucrose they contain, as well as all the other ingredients, including cholesterol, for example. Of course, people in the medical professions, including midwives, nurses, and general practitioners, should all help to promote the prevention message and close liaison between these people should be encouraged.

Detecting decay

Methods of detecting decay early have depended upon a visual examination of the teeth using a dental mirror and probe which catches in any sticky areas. Radiographic pictures are taken to ensure that decalcification of the enamel has not begun at the contact points or, indeed, beneath old fillings. Even when practised by the most experienced dentist and carried out with the best possible care, these methods are not 100 per cent accurate but, no doubt, they will be with us for many years to come. Recently, however, a device has been developed that measures the electrical activity of a decaying tooth which depends upon the moisture content that is present around a carious site. Having taken a reading, the dentist refers to a chart with readings based upon a scale of 0 to 10 degrees of electrical conductivity. A figure higher than 5 indicates that a cavity is developing.

Obviously, X-ray photography will continue to be needed to investigate the condition of roots and bone but, because X-rays are potentially dangerous to dental staff and to patients, it is vital that more stringent regulations should be laid down straight away governing the use of lead aprons and protective screens for the operatives. X-ray machines in use today are extremely well designed and little scattering of the X-rays occurs but there is still no room for complacency. All dental personnel should use radioactivity measuring devices and all X-ray equipment should be checked periodically by the company that installed it or by government-appointed agencies – spot checks are not enough. A recent report, for instance, showed that of 585 X-ray machines in a random sample of practices several fell below the safety standards of the Health and Safety Executive. (Ref. DHSS, Jan. 1979). A certificate of worthiness, we feel, should be on display to show that the X-ray machine in use in a particular practice is safe.

The same degree of priority should be given to the sterilization of equipment used in a dental practice so that there is less risk of transmitting infectious diseases. Autoclaving dental instruments is a most acceptable way of ensuring adequate hygiene but the equipment is extremely costly and this may be the reason why sterilizing equipment by this method is not more commonplace. Again, perhaps the government could assist dental practices to some extent in this important aspect.

Other methods of examining bone and dental tissue may be developed. Ultrasound techniques may have some use in ageing foetuses and recording their dental development. Perhaps we may see a method of identifying the 'at-risk' patients in terms of their susceptibility to dental disorders so that they can be advised on their particular needs for even more stringent oral hygiene.

We hope that dental disease is not in itself a precursor to other illnesses, such as the sore throat which precedes some cases of rheumatic fever. But, one never knows, and there may be a link between some systemic diseases and tooth decay or gum disease. One American professor certainly thought it was worth investigating the changes in blood chemistry that may be associated with gum disease.

Materials science has made vast strides in the last decade. The use of high-impact resins in the construction of dentures and the use of composite filling materials that match tooth colour and have desirable structural properties may mean that the grey amalgam filling and the gold crown can be relegated to the history books.

We have already referred to forensic dentistry but, as decay becomes less prevalent, the identification of human remains from dental records of those burnt in accidents, for example, will become less useful as the pattern of fillings in a given record will be absent. It is important, therefore, that tooth loss in the deciduous dentition is accurately noted in your children's records and that any minor blemishes in the first or second teeth are documented. Of course, this is your dentist's responsibility but sometimes records are lost and a knowledgeable parent may be able to save a considerable amount of anxiety for himself if he knows that, say, the child's second incisor had a deep pit in the surface.

The use of radiography is also important in forensic dentistry and a note in your diary that X-ray photographs of your teeth were taken on a particular day may well prove useful. Tell your family which dental practice you attend and record the name of the dentist that treated you.

It may be that lasers will become more widely used in soft-tissue surgery. Perhaps a silent drill would be of great benefit to patients, dentists, and assistants alike.

Computerization has already entered the dental field and probably, in the future, more and more practices will use them to assist with administration. Their use in research is, of course, most important, and showing the trends in types of treatment within a particular practice may prove to be extremely useful in monitoring the volume and types of treatment in different parts of the country.

Video games using the theme of destroying plaque bacteria have now come on to the market. Perhaps video programmes about dental health could be more vigorously promoted.

The use of fibre-optic light in enhancing the dental operator's field of vision is actually being used already, although it is not commonplace. Holograms have also been used to record orthodontic malocclusions, and this certainly has the advantage of eliminating the storage of plaster models of the jaws – quite a problem in a large practice catering for many orthodontic cases.

It is likely that the way in which undergraduate dentists are taught will change in the future, with more emphasis being placed upon dentist-patient communication techniques as well as on the pitfalls of running a dental practice as a business. Dentists and dental hygienists, too, may be instructed in deaf-and-dumb sign language and, of course, it would be an excellent idea if dental health literature was more widely available in braille editions.

Where patients are unable to understand English, problems of communication can obviously arise. In some cases, community leaders would be well advised to seek information about dental health and arrange for it to be reliably translated into the languages concerned. Sudden alteration in dietary habits can result in dental disaster for some people and they should be alerted to this danger as soon as possible.

We are happy to end on the encouraging note, however, that a survey carried out in 1983†, showed that only 48 per cent of five-year-old children had suffered some dental decay. In 1973, the figure was 71 per cent. Improvements were found in all age groups from five to fifteen years. The most encouraging result was that in six- and seven-year-old age groups, only 19 per cent of children had experienced dental decay whereas in 1973 the figure was more than twice this, at 39 per cent. We are sure that this trend will continue and hope that our book, and others in the same vogue, will assist in the process.

† Reported in *Children's Dental Health*, OPCS Monitor, 1983.

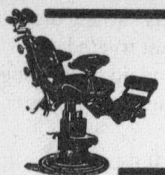

AN AUTHOR'S NOTE FOR THE FUTURE

From the cover on this book, you will have gathered that two authors have been involved in the writing of this book. Obviously, one of us is a qualified dental surgeon and it has been his intention throughout to develop a book which will serve to help people to understand how they can best look after their teeth, in conjunction with a dentist of their choice, and to allay many of the fears which so many of us hold about a 'visit to the dentist'. My own role as an editor and writer has been to assist in that task.

In my childhood, my own teeth, like those of many others of my generation seemed to be an endless source of pain and trauma largely because of a real lack of sensible dental education and, often, misplaced fears.

A persistent image in a nightmare which plagued me throughout my childhood and into my teens was that my mouth would suddenly become overflowing with crumbling, decaying teeth and that I could never find a dentist. I gather that 'teeth dreams' are by no means uncommon and may have no connection at all with dental problems, but it did leave me feeling that my teeth would not last me far beyond my twenties. This fear was heightened firstly by the knowledge that my mother had been fitted with full dentures by the time that she was twenty-eight and secondly because my early experiences with dentists were far from happy ones. One particular incident that I remember only too clearly occurred at the age of eight when my parents were moving house from Wiltshire to North Devon. On the day of the actual move, which in 1957 was rather less easy than such events are today, I was suddenly stricken with searing toothache. Fortunately, then there were less pressures on a dentist's time than there are today and I was whisked off to the dentist that very morning. The tooth was removed; it was a painful experience and I did bleed rather more than I liked although, of course, the socket was plugged with a gauze pad. In this condition, I travelled the hundred or so miles in an ancient Standard 14 motor car to our new home.

Unfortunately, although the bleeding stopped, the pain didn't subside and the whole of the side of my face began to swell. Being new to the area, we did not have a dentist and, over the weekend, my face became inflamed and my temperature rose dramatically. Naturally, my parents were concerned and, on the recommendation of colleagues, telephoned a doctor. To his credit and my eternal gratitude, he arrived at 8 pm on a Sunday evening forearmed with a hypodermic syringe and liquid penicillin. I had a severe infection from the extraction. Ever since I have lived in mortal fear of having teeth extracted not, of course, that I have managed to avoid the experience again since that time. Indeed, I now have only twenty-seven rather than the full complement of thirty-two teeth, most of the molars and premolars are filled with amalgam, and two of them are crowned; a broken front tooth has been restored by acid etching. Not least of my fears has been that I would either lose all my teeth at an early age or that they would be so badly decayed that I would be blessed with an even less attractive appearance than the one with which I was born.

Like many post-war children, I had sugar with everything and, with the demise of rationing, sweets were the new delight to be offered as a reward for all good behaviour. Few children in small country towns were encouraged to visit a dentist unless it was with toothache, and cleaning the teeth was not the standard morning and bedtime routine that it is for most children today. All in all, hardly the best of starts for the health of my mouth and this is the main reason why I was so delighted to be involved in writing this book. Since those early days, dentistry has progressed by leaps and bounds. I actually look forward to seeing my dentist, safe in the knowledge that I can happily discuss the care and condition of my teeth in pleasant surroundings. Consequently, at the advanced age of thirty-six most of my teeth are still in my mouth and look quite good. I now feel very warmly about modern dentistry and look forward to further advances in gum and teeth care.

As a lay person at the receiving end of dental treatment, however, there are still ways in which I could envisage 'the shape of teeth to come'. I hasten to add that these are only the thoughts of an interested person and may not have any place in future reality. From a position of knowledge, the senior author has already outlined the directions that dentistry and dental education may take and from which the public at large could benefit. These are possibilities and probabilities, whereas my own ideas may simply be flights of fancy.

For example, we have already discussed the ways in which techniques have been developed to map the shape of the mouth and its development for orthodontic purposes. We have also looked at the ways in which computers might be used for tasks such as record keeping. Is it possible to link these two developments? Although considerable advances have been made in the materials that are used in taking impressions for denture and crown work, nonetheless, having an impression taken is still not a pleasant experience and does cause some people to retch. The models that result also cause some problems in finding space for storage and, in my case, I was presented with mine to keep at home in case of future need. I wonder, therefore, whether it may, at some time in the future, be possible to map the mouth by means of a hologram and store the record on a computer which could then easily be sent down a telephone line to a computer in another dental surgery should the patient have cause to change dentist. This ought to be less unpleasant and more fun for the patient and be more accurate and efficient for the dentist.

No-one is likely to go out and hire a dental hygiene video tape for home entertainment but perhaps the time spent in the waiting room could be put to valuable use if the room was fitted up with video recording equipment. Provided any films shown were carefully planned and made, the waiting period could be less boring and patients may be able to learn painlessly about the importance of dental hygiene, diet, and so on.

It seems to me, too, that, if it is not already happening, there could be room for greater liaison between the dental and materials sciences in developing new substances for protecting the teeth and for restorative work. We have already looked at fissure sealants, acid etching, the use of acrylics, gold, porcelain, and chrome-cobalt, etc. but one of today's wonder materials is carbon fibre which is flexible, light, and very strong. If it is non-toxic and can be manufactured in the appropriate colours perhaps carbon-fibre dentures may one day be available although, hopefully, by that time, there should be fewer people in need of them anyway if dental education develops in the way that we hope.

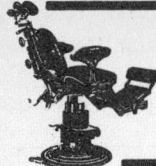

APPENDIX TABLES

Table 1   Dates of eruption of the teeth

First teeth
(Sometimes referred to as the milk teeth or deciduous dentition)

There are normally twenty milk teeth – ten in the upper jaw and ten in the lower jaw. The teeth are identified by the first five letters of the alphabet. The ones nearest the mid-line are the a's and those furthest from the mid-line are referred to as the e's. The arrangement is therefore:

e	d	c	b	a	a	b	c	d	e
e	d	c	b	a	a	b	c	d	e

Average dates of eruption
The incisors (a and b) appear in the mouth at about 7 months
The canines (c) appear in the mouth at about 16 to 18 months
First molars (d) appear in the mouth at about 12 to 14 months
Second molars (e) appear in the mouth at about 20 to 30 months

Second teeth
(Sometimes called permanent dentition)

There are normally thirty-two permanent teeth – sixteen in the upper jaw and sixteen in the lower jaw. The teeth are identified by the numbers 1 to 8. The teeth nearest the mid-line of the face are the 1s and those furthest from the mid-line are the 8s.

8	7	6	5	4	3	2	1	1	2	3	4	5	6	7	8
8	7	6	5	4	3	2	1	1	2	3	4	5	6	7	8

Average dates of eruption

Incisors (1 and 2) appear in the mouth uppers 6 to 8 years / lowers 7 to 9 years
Canines (3) appear in the mouth uppers 11 to 12 years / lowers 9 to 10 years
First and second premolar teeth (4s and 5s) appear in the mouth 10 to 12 years
First molars (6s) appear in the mouth 6 years
Second molars (7s) appear in the mouth 11 to 13 years
Third molars (8s) appear in the mouth 17 years and over.

Table 2   Dental jargon

Surface of tooth	Symbol	Location
Buccal	B	Cheek side of upper and lower molar and premolar teeth
Lingual	L	Tongue side of lower teeth
Palatal	P	Palate side of upper teeth
Mesial	M	Surface of tooth closest to the middle of the face
Distal	D	Surface of tooth most distant from the middle of the face
Occlusal	O	Chewing surface of molar and premolar teeth – upper and lower
Incisal	I	Cutting edge of the incisor teeth, including the canine teeth – upper and lower

e.g. An MOD cavity is one that extends over three surfaces, the mesial, the occlusal, and the distal surfaces

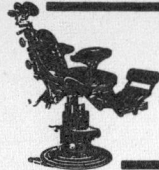

INDEX

Figures in italics refer to captions.

gold filling 54
grinding teeth *see* bruxism
gum 17
  contour of 59–60
  disease 18, 25, 27–31, 35, 42, 49, 52,
      58–61, 118
  recession 61
  'sandwich' 74, *74*
  shield 41

haemophilia 105
halitosis 29–30, 103
handicapped people 103
Hapsburg Jaw 89
heart conditions 100–101, 112
hepatitis 105
hereditary defect 110
herpes virus 107
hologram 119
Homer 94
hydrocephalus 104, 105
hypnosis 85, 98–99

illness 15, 21, 50, 78, 100–113
immunization *see* vaccination
industrial accidents 41–42
infection 81–82
influenza 103
injection *see* anaethesia
irregularity in teeth 84

jaw
  formation 13
  Hapsburg 89
  occlusion *see* occlusion *and*
      malocclusion
  shape 13, 72–74, *72*
  structure 13, 18, *19, 20*, 21, 96, *96*

kidney conditions 105, 109, 110

laser 119
Lavoisier, Antoine Laurent 98
Lee 103
leukaemia 102
lisping 108
liver conditions 105–106, 110
local anaethesia *see* anaethesia, local
loss of teeth 15, 17, 18, 27, 86
lung conditions 103

malignancy 112
malocclusion 22, 61, 84–89, *87*, 102, 119

measles 110
medical history and records 49–51, 98,
      100, 100–113, 118
medicine 46, 49–50, 82, 110–111 *see also*
      drugs
menopause 106–107
menstruation 106, 107
mental handicap 103
mesiodens 90
Mesmer, Franz Anton 98
mesmerism 98
metronidazole 110
migraine 18
milk
  breast-feeding *see* breast-feeding
  composition of cow's and human 44–45
  fluoridation 38–39
  teeth *see* first dentition
mono-amine oxidase 111
monoideism 98
morning sickness 106
Morton, William 95
mouth ulcer *see* ulcer
mouthwash 29, 30, 78, 112

National Health Service 37, 41, 83, 116
nervous conditions 104–105
nervous system 16, 75
nitrous oxide gas 94–95

occlusion 18, *19*, 22, 84
odontome 91
oedema 77
oral hygiene 28, 30, 31–37, 49, 59, 60, 74,
      75, 86, 88, 109, 115–116
orthodontic treatment 84–97, 115
overdenture 66–67, *66*

pain 17, 27, 77, 78, 79, 82–83, 104
  control 94–99
painkiller 82–83
paracetamol 82, 105
periodontal disease 27, 28, 58–59
  see also gum disease
permanent teeth *see* second dentition
phenylketonuria 46
physical handicap 106
plaque 23, 24–25, *24*, 27, 28, *28*, 29,
      30–31, *33*, 58, 89
plate 55, 86
pleurisy 103
pneumonia 103
pocket 28–29, *28*, 52, 58, 59, 61